GOING FOR THE CURE

GOING FOR THE CURE

Francesca Morosani Thompson, M.D.

ST. MARTIN'S PRESS
New York

B-THO

✓

Design by Judith Stagnitto

Library of Congress Cataloging-in-Publication Data

Thompson, Francesca Morosani.
    Going for the cure / Francesca Morosani Thompson.
        p.   cm.
    ISBN 0–312–02921–7
    1. Thompson, Francesca Morosani—Health. 2. Multiple
myeloma—Patients—United States—Biography. I. Title.
    RC280.B6T46 1989
    362.1'969944—dc19   89–30135
    [B]

First Edition

10 9 8 7 6 5 4 3 2 1

To Jim: the wind beneath my wings

GOING FOR THE CURE

SPRING 1986

We fought about it for months. Not the getting sterilized, but who would get the operation. We needed a permanent solution for our family planning. In the last year we had enjoyed an empty nest—Heather at seventeen was a senior at boarding school and going on to college, and J, our fifteen-year-old son, was a freshman at the same school. Although they were home in Manhattan for vacations and we saw them on weekends, because the Taft School is only minutes away from our country house in Litchfield, Connecticut, Jim and I knew they had left home.

Heather was born when I was twenty-four, J when I was twenty-six. Jim and I had never planned for more than two children and felt lucky to have one of each, healthy and beautiful. But I was never ready before to give up the potential: knowing I could have more children insulated me from the fear of losing them in an accident, gave me a handle on the uncontrollable. The years slipped by; we stuck to the old-fashioned, unspontaneous methods. I couldn't tolerate the Pill, the IUD had brought us, delightfully, J, but we thought it was unreliable.

The first year without the children convinced us that we had completed the child-raising years and were unlikely to want to start again. We were enjoying ourselves— eating out on the spur of the moment, going to the ballet and opera, taking ski vacations, studying Italian at night, piano lessons for Jim—doing things we had postponed for years while the children were growing and I was becoming a doctor and Jim was working in advertising.

The decision to get sterilized evolved easily; the method gave rise to arguments. I'll get my tubes tied, I said. Jim objected. I'll get more information. Like most doctors, I gather information in a specialty out of my field by talking to friends and colleagues I respect. What's the best way to tie tubes? "Band-Aid" surgery: laparoscopy with tubal electrocautery (burning) has the potential to burn other structures inadvertently and it can also be nonpermanent. There is a small but definite incidence of tubes opening up again. I remembered a friend who had a miscarriage months after a laparoscopic tubal ligation. Not for me. How about a hysterectomy? Then I wouldn't have to worry about endometrial cancer with estrogen replacement therapy in later years. It's a bigger operation, longer convalescence, and some women complain of painful intercourse, a change in orgasmic response with the loss of uterine contractions. Oh. So what's the best way? A "minilap": a low, horizontal bikini-line abdominal incision. Tubes are identified, about a half inch of tube removed, both ends tied off; general anesthesia, a week off from work. Sounds good to me, except the part about the general anesthesia. Jim cringes: he thinks it would be painful. Why not a vasectomy? Back to my friends. Outpatient surgery, local anesthetic, ice bag for a day or two, take six to eight weeks to produce a sperm-free sample, use other methods till then. Okay. What's the downside? Pause. Well, the quantity of the ejaculate is decreased, some men notice the difference in the quality of the orgasm. Oh.

More arguments, reasons. My reproductive years are nearly over at forty-two, I won't be giving up anything; you are only forty-seven, you have many reproductive years left. So what? What if something happens to me? I would want you to find someone else, you might want children together. No way. Impasse.

I just want it to be me who gets the operation because I'm the one who would get pregnant. Silent assent. I schedule the surgery. A month cooling-off period is required by state law for sterilization. The papers are sent to us, we sign. Even in New York State, a husband has to give permission before his wife can be sterilized. We've come a long way, baby.

I tell my secretary I'll be away for the week of May 19. I look forward to the time off, I've been working twelve-hour days, I'm tired at night. Two weeks before the surgery my teeth begin to hurt, inflamed gums. I arrange a long-overdue appointment with my dentist, prescribe myself some penicillin. No abscess, says my dentist. But he is alarmed at the sudden bad state of my gums. You have bad periodontal disease, take these X rays to a periodontal specialist, you probably need some surgery on your gums. Great, now I'm really middle-aged. Although the painful inflammation abates, I stay on the penicillin because I don't want an active infection to postpone the scheduled surgery.

⋮

SUNDAY, MAY 18, 1986

⋮

We spend the weekend before my surgery in the country, a beautiful sunny spring weekend; the lilacs are out. We leave around lunchtime and drive over to see

Heather and J. I tell them I'm going into the hospital for a routine, elective tubal ligation. J is matter-of-fact. I tell him I'll call him Monday night when I'm back in my room. Heather adopts an ironic, parental attitude, she tells me that what I'm doing is a mature, responsible thing. We both laugh at the role reversal. We say good-bye. It feels like a bigger leave-taking than it should be.

New York Hospital. It is strange entering by the front door on Sixty-eighth Street on a warm, sunny afternoon. Although I haven't been back here in four years, I did work here for nine years—four in medical school, two as a general surgical resident, three as an orthopaedic resident at the Hospital for Special Surgery next door. This is where I became a doctor; now I am a patient. It hasn't changed. I sit with the other healthy, elective surgical patients in the admitting department anteroom. Soon I am called into the small cubicle where the billing information is typed into the computer. Would I like M.D. on my plastic ID card? Yes, I would.

Then more waiting in a room too dark for reading; the light bulbs in the lamps are out. "Escort" will take us to admission testing. All preop patients get basic tests: chest X ray, EKG, urinalysis, blood. Eventually, the blue-coated escort aide ambles in, gathers our paperwork, and guides us to our destination. I follow passively, noting that this is a part of the process of hospitalization I know nothing about.

I undress in a cubicle and put on a gown for the chest X ray and EKG. The EKG tracing is impressive: coded into a new computer, an instant printout emerges—heart rate, axis, PR interval, etc. We used to do this ourselves in the Days of the Giants, i.e, when I was an intern. We cut the ribbon of paper into two-inch squares and taped it into the chart, measuring the tracing with small calipers and recording the interpretation into the chart notes. Now house officers have it easy. I am given a cup for the urine specimen and wait in line for the bathroom. What about the blood work? They'll get that on the floor. So some things haven't changed after all.

The house officer has to do the work of the blood-drawing technician on a Sunday afternoon.

More waiting for Escort, not okay for me to take my chart to the floor, the seventh floor of the Lying-In Hospital. We finally get there. Someone else is in my room, another private room is selected, right across from the nursing station, a noisy place. Jim meets me there, we arrange for the TV hookup.

Soon a medical student comes in with tubes for blood-drawing. He's paying tuition to draw my blood. He's nervous; medical students get very nervous taking care of real doctors. If he makes a mistake, I'll know and judge him harshly. I used to feel the same way. We chat, I try to make him relax. He's class of '87 at Cornell Medical; I tell him I was Cornell Medical class of '77. We talk about favorite professors. The blood runs slowly. I pump my arm. He's nervous again, wondering what he's doing wrong. I say it's probably the vacuum in the tubes. Finally the tubes are filled: violet top for the CBC, red top for the chemistry profile, pale blue top for coagulation studies, yellow-and-red speckled top for the type and cross. I get a Band-Aid and he scurries out, relieved that his mission is accomplished.

Dinner is served, lousy but I eat it anyway. Jim's getting restless. I assure him that I'm fine and he leaves; we'll talk in the morning. My surgery isn't scheduled till early afternoon.

Another young man in white comes in, introduces himself as the chief resident. I recognize the courtesy: normally the intern does the "workup," the admission history and physical; I get the pro instead of the amateur because I'm another surgeon. We get the job done fast, we both know the drill. I anticipate the questions: medical illnesses? healthy as a horse; medications? penicillin for recent periodontal inflammation; surgery? tonsillectomy 1965, benign breast biopsy 1984; pregnancies? G2P2 (two normal spontaneous vaginal deliveries, no other pregnancies); tobacco? stopped fourteen years ago: alcohol? social—wine, beer, Scotch. A quick listen to the chest and heart, a fast abdominal palpation for masses, no scars to indicate previous surgery that could complicate tomorrow's procedure. Job done, he leaves. No problems here.

I decide to call my friend, Anne Moore, a hematologist-oncologist, to let her know I am in the hospital. We have been friends for years. We met when she taught my section in hematology when I was a second-year medical student and she was a young attending. We soon figured out why we looked so familiar to one another—we had been classmates at Smith College.

Anne had gone directly to Columbia College of Physicians and Surgeons; I had married Jim when he graduated from Yale, and we settled in Manhattan after my junior year. I finished my course work at Barnard College, and then earned a master's degree in social work while working at a child welfare agency. Anne trained in internal medicine at New York Hospital while I had babies and worked part time as a casework supervisor at the child welfare agency where I had trained. We met often while I was in medical school; a compassionate, intelligent physician, she was a superb role model and helped me sort my way through the clinical rotations. While I was assigned to the labor and delivery rooms on the obstetrics rotation, Anne and her husband arrived for the birth of their second child. Anne invited me into their delivery room. It was a joyous occasion and forged a stronger bond between us. When I started my internship at New York Hospital, we lived in the same apartment house across the street from the hospital. Our sons, a year apart in age and attending the same school, became friends as well. After I moved away we kept in touch by phone, neither one of us had time to get together.

But earlier in the spring Anne and I had each given talks at a conference for women in medicine. We went for coffee afterward to catch up. Soon after, Anne had been sidelined by some emergency surgery herself, and I commiserated with her during her convalescence. She knows that I was planning elective surgery and will come by for a visit in the morning. Before we hang up I tell her that just in case I have a problem with the anesthesia, like aspirating or not waking up, I want her to look after me for medical problems. Anne laughs, recognizing the anxiety of the preop patient, and says of course.

The evening wears on. I read a magazine. The chief resident pops in with another violet-topped tube for a complete blood count, the CBC. The lab reported that the sample was QNS: quantity not sufficient to perform the test. We both chuckle—residents usually figure that QNS happens when the lab tech drops the tube and loses the sample. The blood flows slowly. He departs with the sample. I watch TV.

Ten-thirty P.M. I'm on the phone with a friend, the chief resident comes in again, waits expectantly. Just a sec, I say to my friend, covering the mouthpiece, and look up at the resident. Is there any reason your crit should be 25? I am stunned. Listen, I've got to go, talk to you tomorrow. I hang up swiftly.

My crit's 25? "Crit" means hematocrit, one of the numbers that make up the complete blood count; it is a measure of the cells that make blood red and carry oxygen around, the red blood cells. Normally, red blood cells make up about forty percent of the volume of blood, thus a hematocrit of 40 is what I expect to have. If my crit is really 25, that means I've got only slightly more than half the normal amount of oxygen-carrying cells; I'm not just a little bit anemic, but profoundly so. I can't believe it.

Also, he adds, your protime is elevated; 17. More bad news. Protime is a measure of one of the blood proteins that modulates the capacity of blood to clot, and a protime of 12 would represent normal blood-clotting, whereas a protime of 17 means I would bleed longer during surgery. Surely this is an error, the Sunday night lab has really messed things up.

These grossly abnormal lab results have to be confirmed. I cannot believe they're accurate, it doesn't make sense to me. I would not operate on a patient who was anemic and had a bleeding disorder until it was evaluated and resolved. These numbers, if true, could mean the surgery has to be put off. Obviously, these tests have to be repeated to rule out a lab error. Out come the tubes again, we send off a violet top and a blue top.

I'm worried but tell myself it's a lab error. A crit of 25 would be equivalent to a loss of five or six pints of blood for me. Acutely, that would be a big bleed. I'd notice that—a torrential period, bright red blood per rectum, vomiting blood; none of that has happened. Not even anything less obvious, dark tarry stool from a moderate gastrointestinal bleed. It must be insidious, maybe a GI bleed so mild it doesn't change the stool color but can give you an anemia if it goes on for a long time; what we call an occult GI bleed. I get them to bring me some hemoccult slides and developer. I produce a stool sample and test it: smear a small amount of stool on a specially treated paper, close the lid of the slide, turn the slide over, open the flap, add a couple of drops of developing fluid, and look at the color. Blue is bad; mine isn't blue. Negative. If I had had an occult GI bleed, I don't have one now.

I call my gynecologist at home to tell her about this wrinkle. She's on her way back tonight from Mexico, says her housekeeper, due in late. I leave my number, ask to be called even if it is late. I want to lobby for doing the operation anyway; I've cleared my schedule and I want to do it now.

I stew. Too late to call Jim, I'd wake him up and what can he do except worry and lose a night's sleep. Besides, maybe it's a lab error. I try to remember what I learned in physical diagnosis, the old-fashioned way of observing physical signs of anemia. Nail beds pale? Look the same to me. I go into the poorly lit bathroom, stare in the mirror, look at the underside of my tongue. Pale pink; too pale? I don't know. I grab my lower eyelashes, careful not to dislodge the contact lens, roll out the lower eyelid. Pretty pale, almost white. Gee, I wish the light were better.

The lab is taking forever with the results. I remember

that it always took a long time to extract the preop labs Sunday nights from indifferent lab personnel when I was a resident, always a hassle because I couldn't go to bed until all the lab values were duly entered into the charts by me, by hand, usually not before one A.M.

Around midnight I figure the results should be down there someplace. I dial 6970, somehow coming up with the number I had called hundreds of times back during my years here. A familiar Islands accent answers. Hematology. I try to sound bored, just doing my job, tired. Is the stat CBC and PT ready on Thompson from M7? Abrupt dropping of the other end, no acknowledgment as usual. I wait, on terminal hold. Finally, Thompson, Fransesca? I hear the mispronunciation and do not correct it. Yes. Rapid-fire numbers. Hold on a sec, let me write this down, but I don't write the extraneous numbers, the normal ones. Just crit 24.6, PT 18. Thanks, *click.* Shit, it's real.

Around 12:30 the chief resident comes in with scraps of paper. Before he can say anything, I say, I know. I called the lab myself. We discuss all the results. Chest X ray and EKG okay, other blood tests, urinalysis normal. No GI bleed by stool guaiac. Chemistry profile pending. No diagnosis.

I tell him my gynecologist is out of town and I don't want to cancel the case yet, maybe we can straighten this out. Let's keep me on the OR schedule, with nothing to eat or drink, so I'll be ready for surgery in the morning. I marshal my arguments: whatever it is is chronic and I tolerate the anemia very well, I work long days, operate for hours, hard physical work; even if it turns out to be iron deficiency or vitamin K deficiency, I could tolerate the operation, which is not expected to produce much blood loss, and we'll work up the anemia later. It's late, he's tired, too tired to argue. He agrees.

I get a sleeping pill, get ready for sleep. The bed is uncomfortable, with no underpad the sheets slip around on the plastic mattress cover. I'm keyed up and exhausted, thirsty but I can't drink—I get nothing by mouth after midnight so my stomach will be empty for anesthesia tomorrow.

Mind racing, searching for a clue. Yes, I was very out of breath when we were skiing in Italy this past February, high in the Alps, seven thousand, eight thousand feet. But we were having a great time, pushing hard, who wouldn't get short of breath at that altitude? We have a wonderful time skiing together. Jim was out of breath too. But hold on, he kept up with me in Italy, was delighted to be holding his own with me compared to our week in Vail in December, when I skied him into the ground and he was dizzy and queasy with mountain sickness the first few days there. And I had been training several times a week all during January on my cross-country ski machine, while Jim hadn't done anything to get in shape. I think about those exercise sessions, how I had gradually changed from continuous skiing to wind sprints, skiing hard and fast for five minutes and then walking around the apartment till my heart rate slowed from 150 to 120 and then back on the machine again, each week increasing the daily distance by a kilometer till I was up to six kilometers a day. I recall a passing thought, quickly dismissed, as I was feeling inordinately breathless: Maybe I should check my crit, maybe I'm anemic.

The sleeping pill takes hold, I sleep fitfully.

MONDAY, MAY 19, 1986

My door crashes open at 4:30 A.M. An aide shoves in, pushing the blood pressure gauge and carrying the temperature machine and a notebook. Vital signs, she grumps.

I'm preop, you don't need my vital signs at this hour. She looks at the NPO sign on the door, warning the aides not to supply me with water or food, notes I'm not the one there last night, departs noisily. I'm wide awake and pissed off. When the other patient switched rooms, somebody didn't pass the word. Shit. My mouth is dry, I'm feeling very dehydrated, very tired, and I can't get back to sleep. The birds are up, chirping outside the window in the gray light.

Too early to call Anne Moore. No one gets up at this hour. Seven would be okay. I don't want to wake them up, but I want to catch her at home before she leaves to round on her patients. Good thing she's a hematologist, just what I need. A bone marrow. Sutton's Law. Willie Sutton, famous bank robber, was asked why he robbed banks: "Because that's where the money is." A bone marrow is where my diagnosis is, fast. In time to stay on the surgical schedule. I picture the stain for iron showing me deficient. No problem.

I try to read, can't concentrate, even on something heavy like *Cosmo*'s Agony column. I long for coffee. Put my robe on, walk in the hall, it's full daylight now. Six-fifteen. Jim should be up. I call, tell him about the abnormal lab test, the anemia. Long pause. What do you think it is? I don't know, maybe I need iron. Do you think it could be leukemia? Don't be ridiculous, sweetie. My white count is normal. I love you. I love you, too, honey, lots. Goodbye, my love, I'll let you know what happens. I'm irritated by his question. Bad disease hasn't occurred to me. Not something that can't be fixed, and soon.

I think some more about what it could be. I remember the chest pain I had when we got back from Italy at the end of February. Sticking, sharp pain just below and to the left of my left breast. Bothers me to breathe, makes me wince when I stand up or sit down, or roll over in bed. Localized to the costochondral cartilage of the seventh or eighth rib. I stop using the cross-country machine, it hurts to breathe hard, it especially hurts to swing my arms back and forth.

Anxious about what was causing it, I suddenly picture a man-eating tumor there. It feels like a fracture. Maybe a pathologic fracture through a tumor. I get our X-ray technician to do a chest X ray on me. I put it up on my light box, study it carefully. Looks normal to me. Fiske Warren, one of my partners, walks in, raising his eyebrows at the unusual appearance of a chest X ray on the wall. We never get chest X rays, we are all orthopaedic surgeons. Is she still here? he asks, noting the breast shadows and glancing into my examining room. No, she's not, I respond testily. Is she you? he asks, picking up on the sharp response. Yes, I admit sheepishly, embarrassed to be caught in my anxious hypochondria over a little chest pain. Now he studies it carefully, too, doesn't see anything either. We shrug. Pesky, but not dangerous, I conclude.

I dose myself with strong anti-inflammatory pills, freebies the drug detail salesman left as samples at our office. After some experimentation, I settle on Feldene, very strong, only take it once a day, very apt to cause gastric ulcers, especially in the elderly. I'm not elderly, not yet, though I'm feeling that way now, moving cautiously to minimize the pain.

After a couple of weeks the pain is almost gone in my lower ribs, but it's superseded by new, acute pain in my left second and third ribs, again at the costochondral junction. I know because I check the skeleton in the surgeon's lounge; anatomically perfect location of the bony and cartilaginous rib where there is a small joint lined with synovial tissue. I have costal chondritis, Tietze's syndrome. A benign, usually self-limited inflammation, no known cause, no specific treatment except time. Could be caused by overuse. I recall the hard skiing, puffing hard. I joke to my friends that I've been making too many obscene calls, breathing heavily into the phone.

I'm relaxed about the diagnosis now, but annoyed by

the disability. Jim and I decide to cancel a trip to Vail with the children during their vacation. Kind of a waste of money if I can't ski, besides Heather would rather see her friends in New York and Jim can take J to Vermont, where my family has a house and I'll go even if I can't ski. I keep taking the Feldene, it helps a lot. Maybe I had a GI bleed back then while I was on the Feldene. That could explain the anemia.

I recall running into a rheumatologist colleague outside my office one day. We chat, he asks how I am, a pleasantry. I tell him about my Tietze's syndrome, get a curbside consult, anything better than Feldene? He offers to do some tests, a rheumatological blood workup, even inject steroid into the area. I picture the needle going too far, a dropped lung, chest tube. No, thanks a lot anyway, I think I'll just let it run its course.

We go to Vermont. I am able to ski, but the weather is terrible, raining actually. We spend half the time reading in the house, a luxurious indulgence for all three of us. The house is high on a hill, the road is straight uphill and doesn't get sanded after some snow and ice one day. We can't make it back in the car after skiing, we have to walk a half mile uphill. I walk slowly in my ski boots and am soon out of air. I complain that Jim and J are walking too fast, what is this, some macho race? I start to cry. Jim takes my bag of groceries and stomps off, obviously exasperated with my temper tantrum. Maybe I was pretty anemic then. Maybe that's when this anemia really began, right after four weeks of Feldene.

Seven A.M. Anne answers, warm and welcoming. Oh, hi, Cesca, how are you doing? Not so great, I think I need you professionally. Oh? pleasantly curious. What's the problem? Apparently, I'm anemic, 25. Gee, that's strange— I'll stop by first thing. See you in a little bit. Thanks, Anne, I really appreciate it.

I get up officially, put my lenses in, brush my teeth,

careful not to swallow any water. I'm very dry. I have a habit of drinking a lot of water, very cold from the tap, two glasses at a time. New York City water is the best-tasting in the world, and the very best, the coldest water runs out of the tap in the bathroom of the nurses' lounge at Roosevelt Hospital, where I work. I wish I were there now, getting ready to do a case, instead of here.

I go out to the nurses' station across the hall. I'm very dry, I tell the charge nurse, do you think we can get an IV started and get me hydrated? She's very friendly and pleasant but says, I thought you were on hold for the OR. Yes, but I'm still NPO, we haven't canceled the case, and I want some hydration soon. My irritation is showing. She stays helpful and accommodating, turfs the problem by saying she'll call the resident for an order.

I retreat to my room, chagrined that I'm acting like a spoiled brat. I wait for Anne.

Eight-thirty A.M. Anne comes in, she has my chart in hand. She looks great, this is the first time I've seen her since her operation. A trim, soft-spoken, pretty woman, a sprinkling of freckles, masses of reddish-brown curls salted lightly with gray, a touch of lipstick, plain gold hoop earrings, understated elegant blouse and skirt under her white coat, kind round brown eyes, an open, innocent face. Kind and soft. A good mommy, a good friend. A doctor's doctor. I've always liked her.

She settles comfortably into the chair next to my bed, assessing me thoughtfully. You look good, Cesca, you look really good. Yeah, but the lab results aren't so good. I start to rattle them off. I know, she interrupts gently, smiling apologetically, I've been studying your chart out there. She wiggles the chart in her lap. How have you been feeling? Well, I concede, I've been tired, but I've been busy lately, operating up a storm, long days. Who wouldn't be tired with that schedule? she responds.

I tell her about being short of breath skiing; I remind

her about the Tietze's syndrome I had told her about earlier in the spring, the normal chest X ray, the Feldene. I tell her about the penicillin for my gums, could I be having some weird reaction to that? It's possible, she says doubtfully.

I remember more stuff; my calves hurt when I walk briskly for a few blocks. I attribute this to no exercise and no stretching for the past three months. Last weekend at a cousin's wedding in Cincinnati I was out of breath dancing with Jim, and my left arm hurt holding it up on Jim's shoulder. We were both a little disappointed that I couldn't dance much, because Jim is a wonderful dancer, and we adore whirling around the floor together. I didn't consider my breathlessness odd, focused instead on the shoulder pain. I've been thinking this was a shoulder impingement syndrome because I've noticed it in the OR, too, when holding a retractor with my arm raised almost ninety degrees. In fact, that discomfort has made me impatient and irritable with the residents I'm helping in the OR. In short, I conclude, I've really been falling apart.

What medicine are you taking? Well, the penicillin. Stopped the Feldene last month. Vitamin B. Why? It's a nice mild diuretic, it seems to keep me from puffing up too much at the end of my cycle, I drink a lot of water. Calcium, a thousand milligrams a day because I don't drink milk. That's it.

What are you eating, are you on a diet? I laugh, I'm always on a diet. Anne laughs, too, and recalls some crazy crash diets I used to go on. No, nothing like that. Just a lot of chicken and fish, fish and chicken, vegetables, fruit, lots of salad, a big salad every day for lunch, from the Korean place around the corner from my office. And beer, and wine, and ice cream—not much of a diet.

Any fevers or night sweats? No fevers, but I do sweat a bit at night, have been for some time, figure I'm just getting close to being menopausal. How long? Oh, a year or two, I can't remember.

Anne does a careful physical exam, looks at my legs for bruises, spends a lot of time gently feeling for a palpable spleen or liver. Nothing remarkable here.

Let's do some lab tests. Sure, I say, but you know and I know that what we need is a bone marrow. I can do it on my lunch break, Anne says. But that's when I'm scheduled for surgery and I want to get this operation done this week, I've cleared my schedule. Anne temporizes, very gently. Maybe we should postpone things a bit, till we figure out what's going on. I have a brainstorm; maybe I could be added on to tomorrow's schedule. Anne goes out to figure out what bloods she wants drawn.

In a few minutes she's back, loaded down with tubes and blood-drawing equipment. Full-court press on the anemia workup, every blood test known, must be with all those tubes. We're rapidly getting out of my depth. Anne smiles, says she'll draw the samples herself, so we can send them off faster. The blood flows slowly, I pump, again. Anne looks at her watch, exclaims with delight, It's only nine, I have time to do the marrow now, let me call my technician, if it's okay with you. Great, I say, the sooner the better.

I sign the consent for the invasive procedure. The technician arrives with a large kit wrapped in blue paper. I remember her from medical school, a great technician and an interested teacher. We catch up on what I'm doing now, across town in private practice with six other orthopaedists, operating at Roosevelt Hospital. Anne tells her I specialize in foot and ankle problems, especially bunions. She is delighted, stops setting up the table, and thrusts her feet at me. Look at these bunions, they kill me! I tell her I'd be pleased to fix them anytime. She backs off, resumes her work, asks how much time she'd lose from work. Two to six weeks, depending on how much time she spends on her feet. She shakes her head, I'm on my feet all day. Six weeks for sure, then. She sighs and says, I don't have the time. Anne is amused, I sense she's heard this conversation before.

We set me up for the marrow. Flatten the bed, take away the pillow, raise the bed as high as it will go. I lie down on my stomach. Sheets are arranged above and below my pelvis. Anne pokes around, feeling for the spot on my left ilium, just next to the sacrum at the base of the spine, where the bone is flat and close to the surface. It's a tender area. She paints me with orange Betadine and announces a little stick with the local anesthetic. It's a hornet bite. Anne asks me to turn my head the other way. I like to watch. It's not that, Anne says, it's just that for some reason there is less muscle spasm when your head faces the other way, and it's easier for both of us.

I turn my head, grit my teeth. Anne changes the needle for a longer one. I'm putting more anesthetic down on the periosteum, the tough skin encasing bone and bringing blood vessels and nerve endings to it. Now for the bone biopsy, a small incision with a pointed scalpel. Now the big trocar, the cutting needle, to bore into the bone. I feel heavy pressure, but no pain. Anne seems to be working very hard, having trouble getting through the hard bone. Do you ever sharpen these? Anne gets through the outer layer of hard, cortical bone and into the softer cancellous bone, where the marrow is. I feel this and it hurts a bit, but tolerable. Anne removes the needle, gives the specimen to the technician, who confirms it is a good sample of bone.

Anne places another needle in the anesthetized area, this is the aspiration, it may hurt a bit. Holy shit, the pain zings all the way down my left leg! Wow! I hope this is it. Anne says yes, and wipes up the blood. Well, I concede, it wasn't as bad as I expected. Anne puts on a bulky dressing, taping it tightly with wide, sticky Elastoplast. You can walk around, Cesca, but not for half an hour. Lie here on your back, keep pressure on it for a while so you don't bleed.

Anne explains it will take quite a while to get the initial results on the smear slide of the bone marrow aspirate, and the bone biopsy will take a day or two. She'll see me later. I tell her I'll get my gynecologist to talk to her. We'll postpone surgery for now and I'll stay here pending plans. But I can have something to drink. I ring my bell, ask for coffee, please, and breakfast. I drink my coffee black, lying back against my dressing.

I call Jim at the large midtown advertising agency where he is a vice president, only fifteen blocks away on Third Avenue, tell him the bone marrow is cooking, I'll call him later when I know something. I lie back, feeling tired and frail.

The phone rings. It's Karen Rosenkrantz, calling to say she had arrived as planned. I'd forgotten all about it. Karen is my cousin, also a surgeon, who recently moved to Boston to complete her surgical training. She's been doing a few years of basic science research in immunology to prepare for a career in transplant surgery; livers, hearts, whatever. She called last week to say she was coming to town and needed a place to stay. I offered her a selection of beds—Heather's or J's. She was supposed to come by my room to pick up the apartment keys. I tell her to come on over. She asks how soon I'm going to surgery. Not yet, there's been a little hitch. I explain quickly about the anemia, the bone marrow. She says she'll be over soon.

My gynecologist pops into the room, bright and cheerful. There was a mix-up with her flight from Mexico, she tells me apologetically, and she wound up taking a flight to Philadelphia and a night bus from there to New York. We discuss my anemia workup. She agrees to do the surgery tomorrow if Anne says it's okay. I imagine she must be relieved not to have to operate today after being up all night traveling.

I go out in the hall for a walk. Passing by the nursing station, I see a woman who used to be an intensive care nurse in the surgical intensive care unit, on F11. We worked well together, and I liked her, and I can't remember her name. She is working now in utilization review, a watchdog administrative job of reviewing charts to make sure people aren't hanging around the hospital, taking up beds for no good reason. Like me, I think. I go back to my room and rest some more. The nurse, my colleague in the ICU, stops in for a visit. We recall funny times, like the time she summoned me from the call room next to the ICU because an old woman was about to have a cardiac arrest in her sleep. I raced over to the woman's bedside just as her monitor showed her heart was fibrillating wildly, hit her on the chest hard, and startled her heart into working again—the old woman never forgave me for waking her up so roughly.

Karen arrives in a white lab coat, which disguises her being a visitor outside visiting hours. I give her my keys. She is mildly but not excessively curious about my anemia and diagnosis. She takes off back to Memorial, where she is finishing up her research projects. I tell her she'll see just Jim tonight or both of us, depending on what happens.

I doze, start thinking back to when was the last time I had a complete blood count, a CBC? Well, 1973 was when I started medical school and then again in 1976 when I had a flu with a high fever for a few days. Too long ago. How about the insurance physicals? About two years ago I got a huge amount of life insurance for my Keogh plan. There must have been a blood test for that. I call our office manager and get the phone number for the insurance man, get his assistant, who says she'll check it out and call me back. I give her my hospital phone number, don't tell her where I am.

Any others? Oh, yeah, I got some bloods drawn in August 1985, after a resident cut me with a dirty knife while I was helping him operate on an infected hip in a drug addict; I wanted to find out if I'd gotten hepatitis. I hadn't, luckily. I call the secretary at the internist's office across the street from my office. I'm pulling my medical records together, can you check and see if you have the lab slips from those tests we did last summer? Sure, just a sec. She comes back, Yes, here they are: a chemistry profile and the serum hepatitis antigen and antibody. No CBC? No, no CBC. Okay, thanks very much—and could you possibly photocopy that stuff and send it to me at the office, please? Sure, no trouble, anytime. Thanks again.

Back to dozing. Lunch arrives, I pick at it, doze some more. The insurance woman calls back. No blood tests were done at all. Really, are you sure? Yes, just the physical, the urine, the EKG, and the chest X ray. Well, thanks for checking.

One P.M. Anne walks in, sits down quickly. I sit on the edge of the bed, she looks stricken. Before I can say anything, she says, It's bad news. What? Multiple myeloma. I leap to my feet, shout, No! but no sound comes out, my throat has shut down. I look away, wail, But we have been so happy together, thinking of Jim, of our life together, crying now. Anne hugs me, I cling, sobbing. It's over, I think, my life is over so soon.

I sit down again. Anne sits opposite, pulling the chair close. How long? I ask. How long do I have? Oh, a long time, Cesca, a long time. She's ducking. How many years? At least four, maybe ten, but we really don't know, chemotherapy is so much better now, it could be a very long time, twenty even. We just don't know. In twenty years I would be sixty-two. Young. Too young to die.

How do they die, people with myeloma?—not me, I mean, I'm not one of them. Not me. Infection usually, Anne says, pneumonia.

I realize I know virtually nothing about myeloma, except that it's the most common primary malignant tumor of bone. Ironic. Bone. My specialty. But we don't treat this disease, oncologists do. Myel-oma, *myel* from the Greek for marrow, *oma* for tumor, *multiple* for the many holes this tumor can make in the skeleton. I think of people with horrendous pathologic fractures, bone totally dissolved by myeloma. Terrible pain, inability to move. Pneumonia sounds better.

I pull away from those thoughts. Are you sure, Anne, are you really sure? Yes, Cesca, I'm really sure; there's no mistake—I looked at the slides myself up in pathology. I remember the rotation I did in surgical pathology, my last rotation in medical school. I know all the pathologists, do they remember me? Omigod, they know my diagnosis, my death sentence. Not only that, I remember the big open ledgers where everyone looks to find the handwritten diagnosis on their patients; they can see my name there, too.

Anne, I don't want anyone to know. Tell them not to tell. Don't tell my gynecologist—she shares an office with other friends of mine, and one of them is another orthopaedic surgeon at my hospital. I don't want this to get out. You know how doctors like to gossip, especially about bad news like this about another doctor, someone they know, someone like them. It's irresistible. Anne agrees to do all she can to keep it secret; we both realize it may be impossible.

You looked at it yourself, what did it look like? Sheets of plasma cells, Cesca, there's no question about the diagnosis. "Sheets"—that's what we say when that's all you can see. Myeloma is a gross proliferation of a special bone marrow cell called the plasma cell. Normally it's hard to find even one plasma cell when you look at a smear of bone marrow cells, only about two cells out of a hundred you see are plasma cells. But my smear is nothing but sheets of plasma cells, I must have it pretty bad.

So what do we do now? You need chemotherapy, Cesca. Chemo? I think of bald patients, emaciated, bald patients retching up their guts. Are you sure, there's no other way? Cesca, you must have chemotherapy.

She goes on, businesslike. But first we need to stage you, find out how much disease there is. Ah yes, I think, the extent of disease workup. My marrow is choked with bad plasma cells and we have to look for more. Hope glimmers, maybe it's not all over, maybe it's just in my pelvis. The first thing, I well know, is a skeletal survey, X rays of my skull, my entire spine, all of my long bones to look for multiple holes in the bone caused by the myeloma.

Okay, a skeletal survey. I don't want to have it here at the hospital. Too many people I know, I don't want to explain why I'm here when they see me on a stretcher. Besides, it's inefficient, they keep the X rays, you can never find them when you want them. Anne suggests an outside group that has a private office in the East Sixties. We send a lot of work to that office, I say, they're excellent, and they know of me, they'd probably fit me in if you call. Maybe we can do it this afternoon. Anne says she'll call them and see if she can set it up. Be sure you tell them it's a secret.

Anne goes on. The chem profile is back, your protein is high, just what we'd expect. How high? Sixteen. That's high, I think, normal range is around 8. All those malignant plasma cells are churning out immune globulin, much more than I need, flooding my body with extra protein. Anne says, We need to check your urine for protein, Bence-Jones proteins. Yes, I remember now, sometimes the kidneys are overwhelmed filtering out these proteins.

You have to collect your urine for twenty-four hours; start in the morning; void, write down the time, collect all your urine till the same time the next morning; we'll give you the bottle to take home. Better make it two bottles, I pee a lot. Good, I want you to force fluids, Cesca, drink a lot.

How's my kidney function? It looks good, Anne responds, your BUN is 15, your creatinine 0.6. That's excellent, I think. Many people with myeloma get kidney failure; I think of dialysis patients, chronic renal failure, what a way to go.

What about the elevated protime and partial thromboplastin time, do I have a coagulation problem? No, I don't think so, it's probably an effect of the elevated protein, throws the test off. What about the other liver function tests? All normal. What about the alk phos? Also normal. Alk phos, alkaline phosphatase, an enzyme that can be elevated when bone is being chewed up by tumor. Maybe that's a good sign.

How's my sed rate? Very high, 150. I am stunned, I've never heard of one so high, not even in acute infection. Sed rate, ESR, erythrocyte sedimentation rate, is a rough measure of active disease. After collecting blood in a black-topped tube, the technician times it to see how long it takes for the red blood cells to settle to the bottom of the tube and form a sediment, what's called the "sinking speed" of the blood cells. When they sink fast, the number is higher, and it's a sign of active disease, although it's not specific for what disease is causing the reaction. A woman my age should have a sed rate of 10, maybe 15. I've seen very sick people with serious infections with sed rates as high as 80 or 90. One-fifty, holy moly, I am sick as shit.

When do we start the chemo? Soon, as soon as the staging is complete. Where? Do I have to come back in? No, we can do it in my office, in the back, we'll bring you right in, you won't have to see anyone. Good. What is it? Oh, a mix of things, the M2 protocol developed at Memorial, it's been very successful. Anne goes on, says she's sure we can get me in remission. Is that a cure? No, the M2 protocol, the state of the art in 1986, has not yet cured anyone. But there is a very good remission rate, at least eighty percent. How long does it take? Probably six months, maybe eight. Then can I stop the chemo? No, you should stay on it for a year—it's controversial, some people would say eighteen months—and then see what happens. Oh.

Anne continues: When we get you in a good remission, we might want to save your marrow, freeze it when it's a good healthy marrow, and save it for later, in case we ever need to transplant it. Sounds strange to me, marrow in the bank. We can talk about it later, after we see how things go. There are all kinds of new ideas, you are so young and healthy, we might want want to consider something more . . . aggressive. Chemo sounds pretty aggressive to me.

Anne says she has to draw another blood test, a quantitative serum immunoelectrophoresis, to measure the exact amount of immune globulins that make up the elevated protein, to quantify the protein being elaborated by the malignant cells. The regular serum electrophoresis was already sent off, it will show an elevated spike; this test is more sophisticated. Also, she'll call the radiologists.

I look at Anne; she looks ragged. This can't be easy for her either, I think, she'll need to tell her husband. You can tell Arnie, Anne, just tell him not to tell. Okay, she says, and departs to make her calls.

I have to call Jim. What do I say? He answers, I echo Anne. It's bad news, I say, multiple myeloma. What's that? It's malignant, a bone marrow cancer. Silence. I start to cry again, hard. I can't speak, gulp for air. Come get me. I'll be right there, curt, short. Then, I love you. He hangs up.

I gather my things, get dressed. I put on the same clothes I wore yesterday, casual clothes, my L. L. Bean off-white pants, yellow buttons-down-the-front T-shirt, knee-high stockings, scuffed brown Tanino Crisci walking shoes. I pack, stuff things in any which way. I move slowly, note a low back pain, radiating down through my right thigh, half-way to my knee. Maybe sciatica, maybe referred pain, not unusual for me, I've had this many times, especially when I'm out of shape. The biopsy site aches dully now, too, on the other side.

Jim arrives. We hug, we cry, sobbing and clinging. There is nothing to say.

Anne comes back in, greets Jim somberly as we pull apart and get down to business. Anne draws the blood for the quantitative serum immunoelectrophoresis. A cheerful young nurse comes in with two large plastic bottles for the urine collection. We try to figure out how to carry them. No room. The nurse goes out to get a shopping bag.

Anne says the radiologists will do the skeletal survey this afternoon, we can go there directly. They understand the situation and are happy to help in any way. Anne wants me to call in the morning, may want to see me tomorrow, wants to set up the chemotherapy as soon as possible, as soon as the staging is complete. I say I'll call her. We leave.

I'm depleted, numb. It's a beautiful sunny spring afternoon. We grab a cab, even though it's a short way. We hold hands. I turn half sideways and study Jim's face as he stares ahead glumly, tanned and healthy, with the same lean, classic features, dark brown brows and eyes, thick long straight hair he had twenty-five years ago when we started dating. He hasn't changed physically at all, and I am dying, sick and frail.

No, think about the good stuff. I give Jim a brief wrap-up of some of the good news. No sign of kidney involvement, alk phos not elevated, whether that means anything or not. I stress the positive: maybe this means we've caught it before something else goes wrong. Anne is sure she can get me into remission with chemo, outpatient chemo, so I can still work, no one will suspect I'm sick.

We pull up to a small, elegant town house on a tree-lined street. The waiting room is beige, modern, nearly empty. The receptionist gives me a form to fill out for the insurance, her boss is expecting me and will be there soon. He is. Nice-looking, tortoiseshell glasses, fiftyish. We haven't met before but have probably talked on the phone, he greets me warmly, ushers me around to the X-ray area, puts me in the charge of a young technician. I change in a booth, we go into a small room and I perch on a stool for the skull and neck views, then go into a larger room where I lie on the table, cold, hard, uncomfortable.

The technician is pleasant, efficient. Chest, abdomen, pelvis, lateral views of the spine. With each view she comes in, changes the large cold X-ray plate, arranging it just right. I lie passively, feeling inexpressibly sad. Tears spill out, run down, fill my ears. This is ridiculous, I think,

like a country and western song parody—*I've got tears in my ears, lying in my bed, crying all night long over you.*

The young woman has noticed my distress and disappeared. The radiologist, smiling warmly, comes in, takes my hand. I don't want you to think we've forgotten you, we're reading your films as they come out, so far everything looks okay, no bone lesions. Thank you. Now we just have to get the long bones, then you can dress, and we'll go over everything together. Thanks.

I pull myself together, take some deep breaths. The technician returns with a smaller plate for my humerus, positions it every which way. It's too short, even on the diagonal. I'm short-waisted, I explain to her, but I have very long arms and legs, especially long arms, I can reach anything on a high shelf, even without tiptoes. She agrees, gets longer plates. We finish up quickly.

I dress. The chief radiologist meets me in the hallway, guides me through a maze to the darkened reading room, lit only by wide light panels motorized to shift up and down with the touch of a pedal. He introduces me to his two younger partners, one of whom I know from our training days at Special Surgery. He scans me approvingly, says, You look great, you've lost a lot of weight since I last saw you. Thanks, that was a couple of years ago, I hasten to explain, nothing to do with this illness. What I mean is, I am not sick, don't pity me.

They get down to business, scanning the boards backward to the beginning. We all look, my curiosity is piqued. It is no longer me on the board, just a patient, a case, and we all know the diagnosis, know what we are looking for: small, punched-out, dark holes where the white cortical bone is supposed to be, any irregularity in the smooth outline of bone.

There are changes on the front edges of the third and fourth lumbar vertebrae, disc space narrowing there and lower down, between the fifth lumbar verterbra and the sacrum. Any old trauma? None that I can recall, but I used

to ride horses a lot when I was a kid, had some spectacular falls. Garden variety DDD, degenerative disc disease, not unusual in middle-aged women with a tendency to over-weight. I think about my low back pain, radiating down to the right. Easy explanation for that.

We scroll the board upward, look at the long bones. I play devil's advocate, ask about the irregularity in the bone in the upper part of the left femur, just below the greater trochanter, the hip area. I know what you mean, says the youngest one, I was thinking that, too, but . . . He squints now, assessing it carefully. Even knowing the diagnosis, he concludes, I have to ask myself what I would call it if it were an unknown, and I'd have to say it's the nutrient artery, totally normal. The others concur. He rolls the board up again, same thing here, indicating the upper part of the humerus, nutrient artery in good bone.

Scroll the board down, look at the lower femora, the thigh bones, and the tibiae, the leg bones below the knee. I scrutinize the right proximal tibia, remembering the pain I had there intermittently a year ago, went away with stretching and exercise. I thought it was pes anserinus bursitis, inflammation in the area where the powerful hamstring muscles of the back thigh insert on the inner side, just below the knee. I guess I was right, they look okay.

Last views are the lower arms. I look at the lower radius, the big arm bone at the level of the wrist. Does that look osteoporotic to you, I ask. Not really; it's hard to say, on plain films, how much osteoporosis there is. Need a den-sitometer, dual photon studies, to really tell. We all know that at least fifty percent of the mineral content of bone has to be lost before it will show on a plain X-ray film.

So the skeletal survey is negative: no bone lesions at all. That's very good. The two younger guys bring up a new idea they've been batting around together. Myeloma is a marrow disease; a new kind of scan, MRI, is turning out to be very sensitive in picking up marrow disease. What kind of test is that? I ask. It's noninvasive, nuclear magnetic resonance. Oh, that, I say, I thought it was NMR. We used to call it that, but it got changed to MRI, for magnetic resonance imaging, because patients were put off by the word *nuclear,* thought they were going to get zapped with radiation, when in fact there's no radiation at all, even less invasive than plain X rays.

Sure, I'll go for that, but it's pretty expensive, isn't it? I recall hearing that one scan costs eight hundred dollars for a fairly small area, a total body MRI could cost over four thousand dollars. Well, this is a pretty interesting situation, I wouldn't be surprised if they do it out of interest, for their teaching files, and don't charge you anything more than your insurance covers. Yes, I say, excited at the prospect of something new, that would be kind of neat, an MRI correlated with the pathologic slides, both before and after treatment. It might even turn out to be a way to follow the disease noninvasively, painlessly. They could write it up.

The chief radiologist interjects, says it's his teatime, would I care to join him while the others make phone calls, check this idea out with Anne, see what they can set up. Thirsty and tired, I say, You're very kind, I'd like that very much, thank you. Thinking we were just going to duck around to an office kitchenette, I am surprised when he leads me up a small back stairway that opens into a large comfortable house—this is where he lives! Dominating the room is a large refectory table; the tables along the sides are loaded with a clutter of mail, magazines, journals; overstuffed chairs here and there; antique Oriental rug, sun pouring in. I feel very much at home.

We settle at the end of the big table near the kitchen, an ample black housekeeper asks if we would like some nice iced tea. Perfect. Homemade. Also homemade lemon pound cake. We chat about the house, the conversion of the office, how fortunate for one to be able to combine the two, work and home, no commuting. I am struck by the amiability of the surroundings, cozy and warm. I would have liked to raise my children in a place like this. Oh, well, not everything is as we would like.

We discuss the X rays, my illness. No, I had no idea I had a problem till today. He is calm, optimistic, tells me a story about a colleague who got a bad-news disease, kept working, defied all odds, still going strong, a reassuring story. Yes, more tea, thank you, it's delicious.

A young man walks in, shorts, no shirt, early twenties. My host's son. We exchange greetings, he joins us at the table, talks about his job or job search, whatever. Finish our tea. I feel relaxed.

Back downstairs. Real world, reentry. Everyone's enthusiastic about the MRI, it can be done Thursday, that's when the machine has enough time available, it may take two hours. My host escorts me back to the waiting room, where Jim looks up expectantly, looking trim and neat in his tan suit. I make the introductions. My host is crushed that he didn't know Jim was there, he should have joined us for tea. Jim, cordial and gracious, says that's all right, he's been very comfortable. I feel a pang of guilt that I didn't suggest he join us, but I had been surprised myself that the tea break was so elaborate. We depart with thanks and go find a taxi. Nice man, Jim says. Yes, very. They're all nice there, they were very good to me.

Home. I fill Jim in on the upshot of the skeletal survey. Very good news. No bone lesions. The MRI Thursday. No, I don't really know what the MRI will show, I've never even seen one. Doing this is kind of experimental, nobody knows what myeloma looks like on MRI.

I tell Jim I'm worried about this getting out. I don't want anyone to know. Don't tell the people at your office, the people you work with. Why? What's the big deal? My practice could be ruined. People don't want to go to sick doctors. They want someone they can count on. Doctors might not refer to me if they hear I'm sick. Might want to spare me. People are funny about cancer; even when they know it's not contagious they're afraid they might catch it. They don't want to be close to it. I say all this, and I have a feeling of failure. If this gets out, everyone will know I have failed. This is the most abysmal failure of my life, a life of success and achievement in everything I've made a real effort to do. I can't say this to Jim, it's too painful to express.

Who to tell? My parents, of course, my brothers and sisters. Jim's parents. The children—but when? Not now, not till school is over, they have exams, they have to concentrate on that. And Heather's graduation, let's not ruin this time for her. This should be a special time for her, a time for good memories, fun parties, a completion. It's going to be hard enough for her to leave her friends, you know how hard separation is for her. Okay, we'll wait till they're home from school. I'm relieved to postpone this, I'm not ready to tell them anything, don't know how to say I may die when they still need me. The ultimate separation. I block it out. Too painful to consider. Let's wait.

My partners, I have to tell my partners, all six of them. They need to know. I may get sick with this chemo, have to stop working; it's business, they should know about it ahead of time. They might have to cover for me if I get sick when I'm on call to the emergency room. It's the fair thing to do. And they are my friends, I feel very close to them. I trust them.

You know, I tell Jim, something like this has already happened in our group, before I joined the practice. One of the partners died a year or so before I joined, he was about forty, I never knew him but I've heard a lot about him. It was very rough on them. He got leukemia about ten years after he was successfully treated for Hodgkin's disease. A complication of the radiation and chemotherapy he had, sometimes it triggers a new leukemia. His last year or so was pretty bad, in and out of the hospital, working, not working. The others have talked about visiting him in the hospital. I can tell it was hard for them to go through that with a friend.

I start to cry again. Jim hugs me. All over again, they have to face this all over again. You know what scares me? What? They're going to withdraw. What do you mean, withdraw? You know, emotionally. It will be so painful, they'll have to back away from me, put some distance between us so it won't hurt so much when I go. That's very common, a natural defense, I say. No, they won't, they love you, and you love them. Yes, I do, that's what makes it so hard.

Dinner—we don't have anything for dinner, and I just remembered Karen's coming to spend the night. I call Chicken Express, something I resort to often when I don't feel like cooking. Order chicken, rice, veggies, salad. To be delivered. The food and Karen arrive around the same time.

What happened? Karen wants to know. Well, we postponed the surgery and are waiting on the tests. No diagnosis? No, not yet, it may take a few days. Oh, okay. Karen settles in, we dish up dinner, nuke it in the microwave. Over dinner we talk about her research, how hard it is to finish up those last details while she's in Boston. Only a month or so left before she starts a second internship in surgery, her penalty for switching residencies from New York to Boston so she could be with Cox Terhorst, who works in immunology at some research think tank in Boston. The commuting relationship was great, but being together all the time is much, much better. She looks very happy, very much in love.

We talk some more about immunology. I confess I know nothing about it, too much has happened since I left medical school. I ask Karen if she knows anything about bone marrow transplants. No, why do you ask? Just curious, I was reading something about it. Maybe Cox does, she suggests.

Heather phones. Mom, what happened? I've been so worried, I called your room and another woman was there and said there is no Francesca Thompson here, everybody's been calling Francesca Thompson, but she left. Well, we postponed the surgery because I'm anemic. Mom, are you okay? Yes, I'm fine, sweetie, I just have to take some medication. Are you really okay? Well, I'm a bit tired; I think I'll rest because I blocked the time out and have nothing scheduled at the office until Friday. Listen, will you get hold of J and let him know what's happening? I can never get through on his phone. Okay—I love you, Mom. I love you, too, honey pie.

We're through dinner. Load the dishes, throw out the plastic containers from Chicken Express. I'm really tired, I announce, they woke me up for vital signs at four-thirty this morning and I am beat. I hope you don't mind, but I have to go to bed. Sure, sleep well.

I am tired. We go to bed, hold each other close. I can't talk about it anymore. I cry myself to sleep.

TUESDAY, MAY 20, 1986

I wake in the early light from a dreamless sleep with a sense that something bad is happening. I wake some more—startled by the realization that something bad has indeed happened. Unable to sleep, I take refuge in the rituals of getting up, then go make coffee, put the instant oatmeal with raisins and spice in the microwave while Jim gets up. We eat breakfast and soon Karen joins us.

Jim leaves for the office, says good-bye to Karen. We invite her to come to Litchfield for a weekend before she starts her internship, if she and Cox can find the time. She says they'd love to. Karen and I settle down with our coffee and tea and talk for a while. She asks if I'm worried about the tests, I seem preoccupied. My control starts to slip; I begin to cry again.

It's a secret, I don't want anyone to know about it. Bad? Yes, obviously. I remember that Karen's father, my cousin and also a surgeon, has recently died of lung cancer, inoperable, after several years of invalidism with chronic active aggressive hepatitis, contracted from years of operating on children's hearts, exposed to thousands of units of donor blood while his patients were on the pump. Karen has dealt with bad disease in her family. I decide to tell her. I tell her the whole story.

I thought as much, she says when I finish. It didn't make sense that you didn't know anything, and yesterday when I first saw you in the hospital, you looked . . . sick, she concludes lamely. Yeah, I guess I am, I say, still not believing it. Look, she says, let me stay with you this morning. I don't have to catch the shuttle till late morning, I'll just call my friend and tell her I can't make it. She phones.

We talk about myeloma, share our shreds of knowledge. What we know wouldn't fill a thimble. Mostly we talk about how it's supposed to be an old person's disease— sixties, seventies, rarely fifties. Not someone young like me. I am struck by the unfairness of it.

On the other hand, it can be fairly indolent; maybe chemotherapy can knock it down and keep it quiet for a long time. I begin to liken it to hypertension and diabetes, dangerous, chronic diseases that may ultimately kill you, but that can be kept in good control with medical management, so you can function well for a long, long time. I feel more comfortable—sure, we can manage this just like diabetes, no big deal.

I am anxious to start the chemotherapy, want to start right now to get this under control. Just like taking insulin. But I'm worried that people are going to find out. We discuss the impossibility of keeping it quiet, but I am determined to try. I don't want everyone thinking I'm at death's door, signing off on me, thinking it's worse than I want to believe it is—it's no worse than diabetes.

We talk about what I'm going to do this week. The MRI, see Anne, maybe start the chemo on Thursday. Ballet tomorrow night. I think I have the energy for that, I love the ballet. This afternoon there's a committee meeting I'm supposed to go to at the County Medical Society. I was planning to play that by ear depending on how I felt after the surgery, so I haven't told them I'm not coming, I might as well go. And I want to tell my partners, one by one. Start this week. Maybe I can catch Bill Hamilton at home after the meeting. Friday I have office hours. We were planning to go to Litchfield this weekend, Memorial Day weekend, but we have to be back in New York Sunday for my secretary's wedding. Are you sure you feel up to that? Oh, I can't not go to that. Ruth would be crushed if her boss didn't come, she's been planning this wedding for eighteen months, it's a very big deal. An all-day event. At least we'll have Memorial Day Monday off in New York to rest up.

And next weekend is Heather's graduation. Dinner for the parents Friday night, graduation Saturday, then we have to move all her stuff. And before that I have several big cases on Tuesday and Wednesday, office hours Thursday and Friday, and some friends are coming to New York and we'll be seeing them Wednesday and Thursday night. It's a lot, I'm very busy, but I want to do it all. We can't let this medical problem get in the way. Well, maybe I'll stop the Italian lessons, Jim agrees we can take a break from that.

Karen has to leave, we tentatively plan for their weekend visit June 7. After she leaves, I decide to brave a look at my old textbooks, read about myeloma. Nothing much sinks in, it's gobbledygook to me. I get that chemotherapy is better, prolongs survival, but there's not much there about how long.

I call our Italian teacher, tell her we want to take a break this summer, maybe we'll start up again in the fall so we'll be fluent again for our usual ski trip to the Alps. She is very accommodating, suggests we might want to just cut back to one lesson a week instead of two. No, we really want to take the summer off.

My mother calls. Your office said you might be home, I'm glad I caught you. What's up? I ask. Listen, I was planning to come to New York tonight, but it turns out Herb is using the apartment. She shares a small pied-à-terre with my older sister and her husband. No problem, why don't you stay here? Are you sure it's okay? Sure, no problem, Karen was here last night and she just left, there's plenty of room. Okay, then, I'll see you late this afternoon, or early evening. Great, see you then. I should change the sheets, I think, but I don't feel like it. I decide not to, Mother will never notice, they've only been slept in once. Good, this will give me a chance to break the news to her.

Going to my committee meeting will get my mind off things. I dress, take a cab to Fifty-seventh Street, attend the meeting. I am able to be my usual cheerful, relaxed self. I enjoy the meeting, a committee of doctors from various specialties who review physicians' charges that the insurance companies feel are out of line, not reasonable and customary.

After the meeting I call Bill Hamilton at home. He is there, as I expect, working on a book at his computer. I tell him I'd like to meet with him to discuss something important, can he meet me someplace? He says his wife is home, too, come on over, it would be fun. No, it's kind of personal and I'd rather see just you. His tone of voice tells me he's now registered that this is serious as he immediately suggests a bar across the street from his apartment, Le Café des Artistes. I calculate how long it will take to get there—no cab at this hour; it would normally take me ten minutes to walk there—I'll meet you there in twenty minutes. I walk to Central Park South and cut through the park. It has rained and everything seems incredibly fresh, lush, clean. I walk along smiling and comment to a passing young woman on what a great day it is. She snarls in reply, totally unimpressed by the beauty of the moment. I walk on as briskly as I can, aware of dull, burning pain in my calves.

Bill is already at the bar, greets me with a friendly pat on the shoulder. I order beer, he takes Scotch. We get our drinks, move sideways down the bar away from another patron for a little privacy. Got some trouble? he asks amiably. Yeah, I respond. Suddenly unable to go on, I stare ahead, unwilling to look at him. I take a sip, shake my head back and forth, trying to negate reality.

Finally I blurt, It's a sad story. Something with you and Jim? No, nothing that simple. I went into the hospital on Sunday to get my tubes tied, I go on, and found out I was too sick to have the operation. I look at him now. He's worried and alarmed. My crit's 25, so I had a bone marrow and it's bad news: multiple myeloma. He swallows hard, eyes glistening with tears, reaches his right arm around me to hug my shoulders. After a few moments we return to our drinks. Shaking his head slowly, he says, Boy, you never know, do you? No, you don't—one day I thought I was fine, and then—this.

We talk about myeloma, he confesses his ignorance of it and the treatment for it. As orthopaedists we see myeloma only rarely in our practice, and that only to do what we can for pathologic fractures and then turn the patient over to the hematologists and oncologists for treatment. I fill him in on the details of my workup so far, the chemotherapy to start this week, my chances of a remission. We finish our drinks and order another round, nibble the goldfish crackers in the little wooden bowl.

How's Jim doing? Jim is—I choke up, searching for the

word—a rock. I don't know how he does it. He says we'll just take it day by day, enjoy each other in the moment. He's always been able to do that, just be in the present; somehow he can just wall off the future.

Who have you told? Just you, so far. I'll tell my family. The kids? Not yet, after they're home from school. What about Ruth? No, I can't tell her, she'd fall apart, and I don't want the whole office to know, just the partners. I tell him I think all the partners should know, it's only right. I want to tell them each myself, I'm starting this week. I ask him not to tell himself till I get a chance to. And don't tell Linda, I don't want the wives to know. Too much chance for them to talk to each other about it, get overheard inadvertently.

Linda's going to be very curious about my meeting you here. Well, make up something, I don't want the wives to know. I feel vaguely guilty asking him to lie to his wife. Tell her I had to talk to you about J, tell her he's been having a little trouble at school and I wanted your advice about how to deal with it. Okay, he agrees, that sounds plausible.

We talk some more about the treatment, the imponderables. I tell him that he can feel free to talk to me about it as it goes along, no secrets, he can bring it up any time.

I remind him that he and Linda are supposed to stay with us three weeks from now. This illness has not changed our plans for the weekend, Jim and I very much look forward to finally getting them up to our house. It's been hard to schedule a convenient time. We have often joked about the difficulties of arranging anything with all of us working so hard.

We finish our drinks, Bill guides me out to Central Park West and hails a cab for me, gives me a big hug goodbye. One down, I think, five to go.

My mother arrives around 8:30 with her small overnight bag. As usual, she's running late. Jim and I have already had dinner and she just wants a snack. We settle on the couch, she talks about how impossible it is to get an early start from Litchfield, so many little things to do. She tried to get off by three, somehow it was nearly six when she left, and the traffic was bad.

I have to tell her, but I don't want her to be upset. Jim takes a chair opposite the two of us on the sofa, pulls up close. You know, a funny thing happened this week, Mom, I say matter-of-factly. Oh, what? Well, I went into the hospital to get my tubes tied on Sunday— Really? she says. Yes, but I didn't have the operation because we found out I was anemic. Oh, just like Mimi, have you been taking that god-awful medicine, too? She's referring to my younger sister, who last fall developed a profound anemia as a side effect of an antibiotic she had been taking.

No, it's not that simple. So I had a bone marrow test—

Is that the test you wanted Mimi to have? Yes, and it showed that I have a tumor of certain cells in my bone marrow, plasma cells, a malignant tumor, cancer. She looks disbelieving. I go on, quickly, focusing her on the positive. I'm going to start chemotherapy this week, my doctor is sure I can get into remission pretty quickly, we've found it very early, it was lucky we caught it so soon.

Mother is horrified. No, not chemotherapy, Cesca, you don't want to go through that—it never works, just makes you miserable. Remember Ned and Nancy? She is talking about my brother John's friend, who died of leukemia at seventeen, and my brother Reto's fiancée, who died of a brain tumor at twenty-six. That was ten or fifteen years ago, Mom, and they had different diseases; chemo is much better now.

I just wouldn't do it, that's all, she says. She goes on, We have to get Lorraine working on this. I grit my teeth in exasperation. I knew this was coming.

Lorraine is what I think of as the family faith healer. My mother is really into all these spiritual things, has been actively seeking cosmic consciousness for as long as I can remember, always the first to get involved in the vanguard of the New Age mystical theories. She spends all her time on this, going to conferences, courses, attaching herself to various gurus. I have always been a great disappointment to my mother, entrenched as I am in traditional Western thought, medical science, stalwartly resisting getting embroiled in the kookier groups, despite heavy proselytizing on her part, although I transiently participated in transcendental meditation, est, DMA—the more mainstream movements. So far I have avoided astral travel, Joel Goldsmith, Rajneesh, Gururaj.

My mother and I have maintained an amicable truce on this issue for years. I don't invalidate her beliefs, and she leaves me alone in mine, however undeveloped they are in her view. All this will change, I know; this illness has exposed a chink in my wall of resistance to things spiritual, and Mother will storm the ramparts to save me.

Mother dismisses chemotherapy as a help, says she will call Lorraine right away, I should talk to her. No, not now, I say. Well, I will, you can feel the vibes immediately when Lorraine gets going on something, it's very powerful, but it's better if you talk to her yourself.

I try to explain why I'm willing to go with chemo. Did you hear this joke, Mom? There's a big flood, everyone flees to the rooftops. There's a man sitting on the top of his house, and a couple of men in a rowboat approach, tell him to get in. No, he refuses, "The Lord will save me," he says. The water rises. Soon a powerboat comes up, he refuses to get in again. "The Lord will provide." Finally, with the water lapping at his feet, a helicopter hovers overhead, lowers a ladder to him, but he waves it off. "I have faith in my Lord, he will save me." The water rushes over the roof, washes him into the floodwaters, and, sure enough, he drowns. He goes to Heaven, meets God, and berates him, "My Lord, I had faith in you, why didn't you save me?" he wails. God responds, "First I send a rowboat, then a powerboat, and finally a helicopter. What the hell do you want?"

My point is clear: I'm taking the rowboat; medical technology is there, and even God would want me to use it.

She backs off. Truce. I know it won't last long. I change the subject. I want to keep this a secret, Mom, don't tell anybody, it could ruin my practice if this gets out. Yes, she agrees avidly, it's not a good idea for people to know, everyone is so negative. It's not good to have all those negative thoughts out there. Let me tell the others, I say, Johnny and Reto, I'll tell them in person this weekend. Don't tell Daddy, she says, it'll really send him into a tailspin. Well, I think I've got to tell him, but I think I'll wait until after Heather graduates. She really wants him to come to her graduation, and he might be too upset to come if he knows.

You're not going to tell the children, are you? Yes, of course I am, but not till they're through school and exams and after Heather's graduation. You'll ruin their summer, I think you should wait until the end of the summer, before they go back to school. Then they'll be busy and won't worry about it so much. No, Mom, I can't do that, they have to know, and I want them to be with us, so we can help them.

.
.
.
.
.
.
.
.
.

WEDNESDAY, MAY 21, 1986

.
.
.

I go to Anne's office at New York Hospital in the morning, lugging the twenty-four-hour urine collection in a small knapsack. It's only a mile from our apartment on Ninetieth and Third; I decide to walk, slowly. Can't get a cab anyway. Notice the low back pain, radiating down into my right leg. It's hard not to limp a bit. After a few blocks I take the bus. Before going into the hospital, I buy coffee for me and Anne at the fast take-out deli I had used years before, nervous about running into people I know who would be pleasantly curious about my being back in the area. I devise a ready explanation: just getting some slides made up for talks I'm giving, just doing some library research. It's true, actually, I do have to write a paper I'm giving in Vail in July at the summer meeting of the American Orthopaedic Foot and Ankle Society. As usual, I've left it till the last minute. I wonder if I'll be well enough to go. What will I say if I can't go? I'm on the published schedule, it's too late to back out. Bill Hamilton can give the paper, he's the second author, he can be my backup.

I find my way to Anne's office on the third floor of the new Starr Pavilion. There's been a lot of construction; I don't recognize it because this building hanging over Seventieth Street wasn't here before. Very posh, lots of polished granite reception counters, no cheap Formica here. The elevators, although new, are slow as molasses, surely a hospital tradition. I've never been in a hospital with a fast elevator; slowness must be part of the building codes for hospital elevators. I avoid eye contact with anyone, don't want to be recognized.

The offices are blatantly marked HEMATOLOGY/ONCOLOGY—what am I doing here?—and some of the other doctors listed there are people I know—they will find out about me and talk! Shit.

Anne greets me cheerfully. Cesca, how nice you could come by, come on in. I brought us some coffee. Great, let's go in back. Her office is an ample corner room, lots of light, modern blond furniture, bright examining room adjacent. I give her the urine collection, she is impressed, Wow, 2600 milliliters, that may be a record. Well, you said to push the fluids. How are you feeling? Okay. I tell her about the back pain and we discuss this at length. I emphasize its similarity to previous episodes I've had, which have always responded to back exercises that I know I should do forever but generally stop when the symptoms disappear—just like most of my patients. We both know there's a possibility this is from the myeloma, agree to keep an eye on it.

How's my calcium? I forgot what you said it was. Normal, no hypercalcemia. Good. Less evidence for subtle leaching of the bones that might not have shown up on the skeletal survey. Anne pulls out the X-ray folder she's already received with a copy of their interpretation. No question about it, they are efficient. It's so much easier to deal with radiologists in private practice, they get the job done well, and fast. We go over the films ourselves, holding them up to the celestial viewbox, the window. Yes, looks fine, maybe a little osteoporosis around the wrist.

We move into the examining room, Anne wants to go over me again. Lungs still clear, good. Pulse 72, blood pressure 110 over 80. Very good. Not really, that's high for me. My pulse is usually in the low sixties, BP 100 over 60. Anne turns off the overhead lights, uses the ophthalmoscope to look at my retina, the fundus, where the microvascular circulation can be seen. The elevated protein can affect these small vessels, which mirror the state of small vessels elsewhere. Like diabetes, I think. Manage this disease like diabetes. All clear. No changes at all in either eye. Good.

I ask whether my blood flows slowly because of the protein. Yes, that's rouleau formation. The red cells get sludged up with protein and stack up, stuck together, so your blood flows slowly, like molasses. It's very viscous. That's when I knew, Anne volunteers, when I drew your blood, Cesca. It's classic in myeloma. I remember when she got the bloods two days ago, suddenly found the time to do the bone marrow immediately. I am grateful. The poor medical student thought it was his fault, thought he was doing something wrong when the tubes were slow to fill.

Anne gets out her prescription pad. I want you to start taking allopurinol. Why? I don't have gout, the uric acid is normal. I want you to have it on board for the chemotherapy. When the cells get killed they release a lot of urate; you might not be able to metabolize it all, we want to protect you from a gouty attack, or kidney damage. Okay.

And you need Pneumovax, have you ever had it? Pneumovax, a vaccine recently developed to prevent pneumococcal pneumonia. No, I've never had that. You should get this, it will protect you. People with myeloma are especially susceptible to pneumonia. Yes, I remember reading that often myeloma presents with pneumonia. I'll order some and we'll give it to you tomorrow when we do the chemotherapy.

Will it make me sick? No, people usually don't have a reaction to the vaccine, just maybe a sore arm. No, not that, the chemotherapy; I have office hours on Friday. I think you'll be okay, any nausea you might have should be at night if we do it in the morning, and I'll give you some Compazine.

So what poisons are we going to use? I mean medications, but it's hard not to think of chemo as poisoning. Anne lets that slide, responds positively: It's the M2 protocol, five different agents, all effective against myeloma cells. Two you take by mouth—prednisone and Alkeran, also called melphalan. That's okay, I'll call it Alkeran, melphalan is hard to pronounce. I'll write you a prescription for those and you can get them over on Third Avenue, they're very nice there and have the best prices. If you'd like I'll ask them to deliver it here for you and they'll send you the bill. That would be more convenient.

Anne goes on: Three will be IV, we'll do that right in here, and also hydrate you with a liter of saline so you tolerate it better. What are the other three? Vincristine—I'll only give you half the usual dose of that because of peripheral neuropathy problems, that's what we usually do with surgeons. We don't want you to lose the use of your hands, that wouldn't be fair. Oh, yes, I think, let's be fair in all this, struck again by the unfairness of it.

Also Cytoxan, it's very good with myeloma, and

BCNU. I remember BCNU; when I was a resident, we used to call it "Be Seein' You." We didn't expect to be seeing those patients for long. Now I'm one of them.

Anne interrupts my thoughts. Cesca, you better get a wig, your hair might fall out with this. Startled, I picture myself with no hair for Heather's graduation, wearing some wig. How mortifying. Close to tears, I say, How long will that take, will I still have my hair by next weekend? Oh, yes, that should be okay, and it may not happen at all, you might not lose your hair at all, different people react differently, some just notice some thinning that no one else could notice. Well, at least I have pretty thick hair, I say grimly. Where do I go for a wig? The nurses have a whole list of places our patients have used and we'll give you a copy. Good, maybe I can get one tomorrow.

Someone ought to come with you tomorrow, can Jim do that? Yes, he's planning to. We're going for the MRI first thing, then we'll come over here, if that's okay with you. That'll be fine. Before you go, Cesca, we have to get your weight and height so I can calculate the doses to order, we do that by weight. I laugh. In that case, I think the doses will be very large. Anne shares my amusement but demurs, You're not fat, Cesca, just big. Do you think I'll lose weight? I ask hopefully. No, I don't, in fact, maybe just the opposite. I think of the steroids, prednisone. Do you think I'll blow up? I think you'll have to watch it. And you should give up alcohol. What? I like my wine and beer. Well, it would be better if you stop, and we'll see how things go.

Anne has to see another patient, turns me over to the nurse, I say I'll see her tomorrow. The nurse takes me over to the scale, right out there in the open, how embarrassing. I hate being weighed, especially on old-fashioned doctor's scales. It's hard to cheat, can't lean around and find the lightest reading the way I do on my own scales at home. I empty my pockets, remove my belt and shoes. Shit, I've gained weight. Eight to ten pounds, sure sneaks up fast. And I've shrunk, not quite five nine—I used to be five nine and a half. Well, everybody shrinks a bit as they get older; the disc spaces dry out, collapse down.

I take a cab home, lucky to catch one right outside the building where someone is getting out. Stop at a pharmacy near home and get the allopurinol, go home to rest.

In the afternoon I call Fiske Warren at the office. I had previously told him of my plans for the tubal ligation, so he assumes I am recuperating at home. We chat for a while, I ask him if he's going for a run as usual after office hours. Yes. I suggest he could end up at the Engineer's Gate on Ninetieth Street and come over for some hydration while he cools down. Okay, but I'll be in running clothes, he says apologetically. That's okay, I'm just wearing shorts myself.

Fiske arrives around six, out of breath and dripping with sweat after six miles in about forty minutes. He drinks two huge glasses of water at the kitchen sink. I get him a large beach towel to wrap up in, get out a couple of beers. These may be my last beers for a while. We settle on the couch in the living room.

He starts to talk about baseball, our usual and favorite topic, endlessly dissecting the players, the plays, the standings. I am the learner, hooked on baseball this year, the first time I've ever had the luxury of time to get involved in baseball, a glorious time sink. The Mets are doing well. Fiske is Jim Parkes's assistant as orthopaedist to the team, covers half the home games out at "the Yard," Shea Stadium. Earlier in May, I went to my first Mets game with Fiske. We had dinner in the press cafeteria, sat with Jack Lang, the sportswriter for the *Daily News*. Watched the game in the "family box," a booth on the fourth floor. Stopped by the radio broadcast booth and met Bob Murphy and Gary Thorne. Checked in at the trainer's room, where medical stuff is handled, where Gary Carter gets his right knee taped before every game, standing on the examining table, head sticking up through a hole in the ceiling where the acoustic tiles have been removed to give him room. Went downstairs to the field level, stood at the gate where the radar gun clocks the speed of the pitches, protected by a thick plastic window from foul balls careening into it with a loud crash. The Doctor, Dwight Gooden, was pitching. Only 88 miles an hour, not his fastest stuff. I couldn't even see the ball.

I change the topic abruptly. I have to tell you something, Fiske. I have his attention. It's a sad story. I didn't have the operation. I was too sick to have the operation. Quickly, I go on; it's easier to get it out this time. My crit was very low—25—so I had a bone marrow and—now I start to cry again—I have multiple myeloma. Fiske is speechless, eyes red, pulls me onto his shoulder. I cry some more, struggle for control, embarrassed to be such a bad sport. I grab my beer, finish it, head off to the kitchen for another. I'm moving like an old woman, I say, noticing my posture in the mirrored wall. No, you're not, you look good, Fiske counters. I return to the living room with two beers. My sed rate is 150, I say, further documenting this illness, assaulting his disbelief. He knows as well as I do that that means this is bad.

More talk of the test results, the planned treatment. I tell him not to tell, hard as it is. Don't tell Michelle. I go over the same ground I'd covered with Bill. Nothing more to say about it, we change the topic, seeking relief in baseball, always interesting.

I notice the time, announce I'm going to the ballet tonight. Good, Fiske says. I'm meeting Jim there, going to take a cab, want me to drop you off on the way? Sure. I surprise him with the speediness of my change from casual to dressy clothes.

We go downstairs, walk out on the street, eyes out for a passing cab. Fiske suddenly realizes he's left his keys upstairs. We turn back, walk fast uphill. By the time we are in the elevator, I am puffing, totally out of breath, calves aching again. I give my keys to Fiske so he can run ahead and retrieve his keys, I can't keep up. He meets me back in the hall and we go out and this time find a cab right outside the apartment. Our cab goes across Seventy-ninth Street, Fiske offers to get off on Park, jog home from there. We say good-bye, he darts out into traffic, off and running, looking distraught. I hope he's not too distracted to notice the traffic. Two down, four to go.

The ballet is *Midsummer Night's Dream*. Jim enjoys it. I am lost in my thoughts, fall asleep. We leave at the intermission. I'm exhausted.

THURSDAY, MAY 22, 1986

Jim and I take a bus to Seventy-second Street, find the office for the MRI in a beautiful new building near the East River. I fill out the insurance forms, use Frances Thomas for the name to be printed out on the computerized identification on every image. It's okay with me for this MRI to be used for teaching purposes, but not with my real name on it. The technician greets me, a young, red-haired, freckled, friendly guy who looks like a teenager but is probably in his twenties.

He explains that any metal would throw off the magnetic field that is used to create the images, so I must remove all my jewelry and any underwear with metal. I change into a gown and robe in a small booth, put my earrings, necklace, rings into my purse, lock all my belongings into the booth, and give the key to the technician. I follow him into the large shielded room that houses the MRI machine. The machine looks like a CAT scanner, with a sled that slides the patient into a large cylinder. I lie on the padded sled, scrunching down to fit my shoulders and arms into the shallow cavity. All set? the tech asks. No metal? Yes.

He hands me some cotton for my ears, to dampen the sound generated by the machine. I stuff it in, he speaks loudly so I can hear. The first thing is to calibrate the machine, there is a loudspeaker and I'll tell you what we're doing from the control booth. He nods to indicate the glass-walled end of the room where the computer console and image screens are housed. I can hear you, too, so let me know if there are any problems. I nod okay.

He slides my upper body into the cylinder. It feels close and dark. Good thing I don't have claustrophobia, I think, feeling confined nonetheless. The tech retreats to the control booth and soon I hear a sound of distant drums, which becomes louder, closer, enveloping me. The natives are restless, I muse. No, sounds like the bass line of a heavy metal group. Suddenly the sound stops. The tech comes in and makes some adjustments on the cylinder, adjusts the position of the sled, says he'll start the first scan, explaining that the machine can only scan a small area at a time. It'll probably take about eight passes to do the whole body scan. Each scan will take ten to fifteen minutes, but I must not move a muscle.

I lie in the shadow of the scanner, listen to the insistent beat of encompassing sound, become mesmerized by it. Time passes swiftly, it's not as boring as I'd thought it would be. Every so often, the tech returns to change the sled position. I notice some other men in the control booth, alarmed that I recognize the head of radiology at Special Surgery. I duck down, hope he doesn't see me.

Finally the scanning is finished. I look out, the coast is clear. I change back into my clothes and return to the control booth. I meet the radiologist who set up this scan the other day. We haven't met before, but he is friendly, interested, and readily agrees to show me the images just generated. I tell him my husband is very interested in computers, can he watch, too? Sure. I get Jim from the waiting room.

The radiologist explains the technology of the scan. It's very complex. Basically, the machine generates a radio signal that bounces off the protons in the nucleus of each atom, causing them to spin in the same direction briefly; when the signal stops, the protons slow down at varying speeds, depending on the size of the atom of which they are a part, and send back an echo that is picked up by the scanner. The computer software interprets these echoes according to complex mathematical formulae and creates images of the relative density of the stuff sounded. Black is hard, white is soft, and the grays are in between. The images generated are aligned as crosswise sections of the body, like salami slices, or lengthwise slices, like a split banana. I don't understand it at all, but the pictures are astounding to me as a surgeon, the anatomic representation is like a black-and-white photograph of a cadaver dissection. It really is a thrill to see this for the first time.

Back to cases—my case. We look at the scans, crosswise and lengthwise, and I focus on the inside of the bones. The hard cortical bone is black, the marrow inside is gray and should be a homogeneous color. It isn't. It is mottled, light and dark gray, all over. Not just in the pelvic bones where the major blood-forming marrow lives, but all up and down the long bones too. I realize I had been hoping that my myeloma was somehow confined to a small area, was just an isolated finding. The truth is plain to see, graphically illustrated in mottled gray: I am riddled with disease. I look from the screen to my arms and legs, realize that my bones are packed with malignant plasma cells. Getting rid of them seems impossible.

I quash these thoughts, focus on the picture on the screen, a lengthwise longitudinal slice of thigh, forward of where the femur is, where the quadricep muscles are depicted in exact anatomic detail. What's that? I ask, pointing to light gray shadows on the edge. That's—uh—adiposity. I laugh. Oh, fat, I guess I have plenty of that.

We conclude our review. The radiologist says he'll dictate his report later and send copies of the scan to Anne. I point out the misspelling of Frances as Francis, which will look odd on images of a female patient. No problem, that can be corrected easily. I wish the marrow signal could be corrected as easily.

Jim and I walk the two blocks to New York Hospital, stop at the hot dog stand for a quick lunch. Fuel up before chemo, Anne had said it goes better if you're not hungry. I skip the sauerkraut, though.

Anne is warm and welcoming, as usual. She ushers us into the examining room in back, says we can do it here, she doesn't need the room, and we'll have more privacy here than in the group chemo room, where outpatient chemo is usually administered by the chemo nurses. A nurse comes in to start the IV, draws a CBC while she's got the butterfly needle in the vein, then hooks up the saline. Jim looks away, he's always been squeamish about blood.

Anne comes in with two syringes of chemo and a small IV bag. The BCNU and the vincristine will go in by IV push, the Cytoxan by IV drip, gradually. She hooks these into the IV line, pushes each in slowly, asks if I notice any funny taste or smell. No, nothing, why? Well, some people comment on it. She connects the small plastic bag to the tubing, hangs it higher than the bag of saline, adjusts the microdrip to a very slow rate. Just lie here and rest while this runs in, I want it to take at least a half hour. We'll be right outside, be sure to let us know if you feel any burning in your arm.

Before leaving, Anne gives me a booklet on chemo to read, *Chemotherapy and You: A Guide to Self-Help During Treatment,* published by the Public Health Service of the National Institutes of Health. It looks simpleminded, with big illustrations of happy, relaxed people, like a child's reading book. I read it avidly, I need all the help I can get. I learn that it would not be a good idea to get pregnant during chemotherapy, the anticancer drugs could damage the baby. No shit, Dick Tracy. Also, my medicines are designed for me alone, and I shouldn't give them to a friend, or let small children get hold of them. This is a big help.

I skip to the meat of the matter, the back section that lists all the drugs commonly used, and their usual side effects. I circle my five, and read about them, alphabetically. I wonder if I really should do this, maybe I'll develop the side effects I read about. Nonsense—I'm not that suggestible, am I? I scan rapidly, this reads like the *PDR,* the *Physicians Desk Reference,* where everything bad that can happen is listed to the point that no sane person would take any drug. Fever, chills, mouth sores, GI bleeding, bruising, jaundice, cessation of urination, cough, joint and muscle pain, abdominal pain, palpitations, dizziness, face and foot swelling, sore throat, shortness of breath, weight loss, hallucinations, blurred vision, headache, agitation, bed-wetting, depression, weakness—all these deserve medical attention. No kidding. Problems not requiring medical attention are few: nausea, vomiting, hair loss, and false sense of well-being. Hey, I could use some of that false sense.

There's nothing here about how the drugs work. I try, unsuccessfully, to remember where it is that chemo works on the cells. Is it in mitosis, when they divide? Where do the dead cells go? No answers here.

I retreat to the Dick and Jane part. Drink a lot of fluids, shower every day, stay out of the sun, avoid alcohol, get enough rest, eat balanced meals, don't cut yourself. Yes, Mommy, I'll be very good. I can't read the part about losing my hair, that makes me cry. I give the booklet to Jim, trade him for *The New York Times,* get lost in the sports pages.

The little bag is empty, it'll take forever for the rest to go in at this rate. I open the IV up all the way, still a slow drip with the microvalve on. Anne comes in with a little brown bag from the pharmacy, my new pills. She writes down the schedule of pills. The Alkeran comes in 2-milligram size, take two in the morning and two at night, there's a total of twenty-eight pills for the week, that's all for this cycle. The prednisone is in 10-milligram size, take 60 milligrams a day for a week, then 30 milligrams a day for a week, then 10 milligrams a day for a week, then 5 milligrams a day for a week, then stop.

That's a huge amount of prednisone, I object, and for a long time. I don't want to knock off my hip bones. In my work I have seen many cases of aseptic necrosis, dead femoral heads, as a result of steroid use, especially high-dose use over a protracted period, which ends in crippling hip arthritis and, ultimately, prosthetic hip replacement. I wouldn't be able to ski anymore. All the bad things I just read about are as nothing to me compared to this. I picture my partners fixing my hips, which prosthesis to use, cement or no cement, all unanswerable questions in a young person like me. I want no part of it. Anne temporizes: I don't think it will happen to you, not with this dose, and on the next cycle we'll use even less, and taper more rapidly. And, she emphasizes, prednisone is very good against myeloma cells. That is the main priority for now. I have to agree, albeit reluctantly.

What about a stress ulcer? Prednisone can do that too. We used to put people in the ICU on cimetidine as prophylaxis so they wouldn't get stress ulcers, how about my taking some of that? Any problem with the chemo? No, that's probably a good idea; I don't think it would hurt, and it might help. I've heard there's a new cimetidine that you only have to take twice a day instead of four times, which one is that? Zantac, that would be fine, I'll give you a prescription.

No need, I'll just order it from my pharmacy.

Anne hands me a third bottle. This is Compazine, for nausea. I want you to take one today at three, so you won't feel sick tonight. Okay, but do you think I'll really need it? Perhaps not, but just in case, I think you ought to take it.

Next week I want to see you in the office. I think about my schedule, how's Thursday? Fine. Now this weekend I'll be off but one of my associates will be available and I want you to call if you have any problems, especially fever. I'll tell him about you, but he will keep it quiet, you don't have to worry about that. And drink a lot of fluids, but no alcohol.

Anne bids us good-bye, asks me to wait for the nurse, who will give me the Pneumovax shot and take out the IV when it's done. I pull out the list of wig shops I'd picked up the other day. We select a place on Fifty-seventh Street, not too far from my office, and not that far from Jim's. I want to get a wig and then go to the office and talk to Drew Patterson, my senior partner. Jim wonders if I can handle that. Sure, I feel fine, and I'm sure you have stuff you need to do at the office when we finish at the wig store. I need Jim there for moral support when I try on wigs.

The IV is finally finished. The nurse comes in, gives me the shot, and removes the IV. I feel fine, rested, no queasiness even. We take a cab to Fifty-seventh Street.

The wigs on view are ghastly, punk styles with orange spikes, Dolly Parton platinum wigs. I don't see anything normal-looking on view. I tell the saleswoman that I'm looking for something that looks just like my hair, do they have anything like that? Of course, please sit down. We study my hair color: sandy blond with quite a lot of gray, especially in front. Do you have wigs with different hair colors, with gray mixed in? Oh, yes, indeed. She selects several small boxes, opens them. The wigs look like little dead animals, squished in the box. She shakes them out, fluffs them up. We hold them against my hair, finally find a color that's a pretty good match, perhaps a little more mousy brown, a little less gray than my own.

I try one on. I am dismayed. It feels and looks like a

lamp shade perched on my head, totally ridiculous. I could go on *The Carol Burnett Show* as her mother. Jim is suppressing laughter. Near tears, I explain that I've just started chemotherapy and I want something that's going to look just like my hair, my color, my style, everything. She explains that they have many styles, she'll get a shorter, more youthful style. I try it on, still too much volume, too long, we decide. A shorter one, this is more like it. But it still doesn't look like my style. She hands me a brush, tells me to brush it around like my own hair. I immediately stroke it askew. No, just light, shallow strokes. I try again. A little better, but still too much volume. She gets another one, even better. I work on this one.

If I want to get this one, they can make it even better by trimming it to match my style. What's it made of? Dynel, a synthetic. How do you clean it? Just soap and water, the directions are in the box. How much? A hundred seventy-five dollars. Okay, I'll get it. Another woman comes over with scissors, and we collaborate on a judicious trimming, getting it to take on the shape of my own hair. While we're doing this, the saleswoman takes my American Express card to ring up the sale. Don't leave home without it. The wig is placed in a large old-fashioned hatbox. I put the chemotherapy book inside too. Before leaving, I get a drink of water from the saleswoman and take the Compazine pill.

Jim takes off for the office, I find a pay phone. I want to talk to Drew, who should be having office hours now, but I don't want to go over to the office unless he has time to see me. Drew's secretary puts me right through. Hi, he says warmly. I get right to the point, tell him I'd like to talk to him. He immediately says he has to drive one of his patients, a friend from Bronxville, home, and he wouldn't be able to stop by my apartment for a drink on the way. I'm close by the office, I respond, I was thinking of coming over now if he has time. I have all the time in the world, he says, see you soon.

On the way to the office on Fifty-eighth between Eighth Avenue and Columbus, I think about what he said. Very strange. Why did he assume I was going to ask him over for a drink? He knows, I conclude. The secret is out, Bill or Fiske told him. I don't like it, I'm pissed off. I wanted to tell him myself, have some control over the information getting out about me. Also, I feel a little guilty. I should have told him first, but the timing wasn't right, he wouldn't have been in the office late Tuesday afternoon and he's never in the office on Wednesday. But still, he's our senior partner, the glue that holds all seven of us together with his absolute fairness and integrity, his sensitivity to all our needs, and I probably should have told him first, before he heard it from someone else.

Drew is between patients when I arrive at the office. I sit down across from his desk, he closes the door and sits down, looking at me expectantly, interested. I have the feeling that you already know what I came here to tell you. Yes, he says, sympathetic and sad, yet very together. Fiske told me this morning after conference. I am sorry, I say, I wanted to tell you myself, I should have told you first. No, that's okay, I'm glad you didn't, it's given me time to think about it before talking to you. Don't blame Fiske, he was so distressed. He came late to conference, looked like hell, he just had to talk to someone about it, and he knew you were planning to tell all of us. I remain silent.

You know, Drew goes on, I've been thinking about this all day, and I think you might want to reconsider telling the others. Why? Well, simply, if we want to keep this a secret, which is probably a good idea, then the fewer people who know about it the better. Also, if rumors get out, people will ask the others if it's true. If they get asked, they will be much more convincing if they know nothing about it. At least until we see how it goes. We have no idea right now what's going to happen. Thats true, we don't, I say. I just started chemo today, and Anne Moore thinks I'll be able to keep working, thinks I have a very good chance of achieving a complete remission, there's only a very small chance that I'll have to go in the hospital on this protocol. But maybe we'll do something more aggressive later.

I can stonewall it, Drew says. If someone asks me about you being sick, I can just say it would be a surprise to me, point out that you're in the office every day, seeing patients, operating up a storm. Why don't we just keep it like this until the dust settles. Bill and Fiske and I know, and that's the bulk of the senior partners, and we'll just hold off on the other three. Don't you think they might feel betrayed, left out, when they find out later? No, I don't think they will, and if they do, I'll talk to them, tell them it was my idea, they won't be mad at you. Okay, I say, let me think about it.

You know, Drew goes on, if it comes to you needing to be out of work for a while, the partnership agreement provides for that. We are self-insured for the first six months of disability, so you will get your regular salary and draw, I don't want you to worry about that. Yes, I remember the agreement, that's very nice. But I hope I won't have to take any time off. I want to keep working.

What about the call schedule? Drew asks. I can cover you, maybe switch some weekday nights that aren't so bad for a weekend call, so you can go up to Litchfield and rest. No, thanks very much, but I want to stay on call, it's not very often anyway. I feel moved by his offer but very much don't want to be vulnerable. I can't stand the idea of not doing my share, no matter what. This is no time to crump out. I want to be healthy, and to do that I know I must act healthy, keep doing everything I always do. I'm sure I can do it if I want to enough, and I want to, a lot.

I get up to leave, Drew walks me to the door, reminds me that he'll be available if I change my mind about the call schedule. His secretary asks me how my vacation has been. Oh, nothing special, I improvise, just running back and forth between Litchfield and New York, doing stuff that has to be done. She says she'll see me at Ruth's wedding. Cheerfully, I respond, Yes, I can't wait, it'll be the event of the year, it's been so long in the planning, Ruth's been a nervous wreck about it, I hope it all comes off well. Inside I dread this wedding, afraid I'll have to stay so long my fatigue will show, and I don't feel much like celebrating.

I take a cab home and remember that my nephew is having his fourth birthday party in my building that afternoon. My sister-in-law had asked me to stop by the third-floor terrace of our mutual apartment house, where large, noisy parties can be held just next to the laundry room, a good place for twenty or thirty four-year-olds. Good thing it didn't rain, imagine all those monsters in one small apartment. I arrive as parents are collecting overtired children clutching their party goody bags. Good, it's almost over.

I sit down next to my mother, realizing I am totally spaced out, a zombie. Why do I feel so strange all of a sudden? Compazine, that's it. I hope this doesn't last long, I don't like feeling disconnected. I tell my mother I don't feel so hot, no, not nausea, but the pill I took to prevent nausea has really zonked me out. I decide to go home, just a ride up the elevator. I escape with excuses about fixing dinner.

At home I decide I have to get organized with all these pills. I pull out Anne's schedule of prednisone and Alkeran, write the initials of the pills in my little red diary, my portable brain, where I keep all phone numbers, my schedule, all relevant bank numbers. I'm lost without it. There, now I won't forget, I'll just cross off the initials when I take each pill: allopurinal, Zantac, prednisone, Alkeran in the morning, prednisone at noon, Alkeran and prednisone at night.

Anne calls me at home to ask how I'm doing. Fine, except this Compazine is terrible, I'm totally out of it, I won't take it again. She is sympathetic, says I must be unusually sensitive to it, most people don't feel so strange with it. She reminds me to keep in touch if I have any problems at all, otherwise she'll see me next week for a checkup and some blood tests.

I get up first on Fridays, at six, because I have to be out of the house by 6:40 to get to the hospital by seven for my weekly teaching conference with the residents. I feel okay, no nausea at all, but I don't feel like lugging my slide projector down there, so I'll talk about sprained ankles again. The interns and residents rotate every month or so on our trauma service, and I orient my sessions to the interns, going over the basic things they need to know, assuming they didn't learn this in medical school any more than I did. When I was an intern and resident, I often felt I was expected to have been born knowing about certain problems, and it took me quite a while to figure out things that are really simple and could have been easily explained if anyone took the time. Sprained ankles were one of those mysteries. The residents seem to enjoy the sessions, even stay awake and ask questions.

After the conference I while away the time till office hours in the surgeons' lounge, reading the paper and chatting with my colleagues. Today I skip the coffee. I don't know how many cups of coffee I drink, it's too numerous to count. Coffee and prednisone are a potent combination for gastric ulcer creation, and I resolve to limit myself to one, at most two, cups a day. In the office I'll brew decaf. I hope I don't get a caffeine withdrawal headache.

I start in the office at nine. Earlier than usual, but I have a lot of postoperative patients to see after being away all week, and I'm ending the day at lunchtime because it's Memorial Day weekend and Jim's office is closing early, we want an early start to Litchfield. Things run smoothly, I don't get behind even though I'm heavily booked: seventeen postoperative follow-up patients and two new patients. A big day in itself, but squeezed into four hours. I enjoy myself; I like changing dressings, get tremendous satisfaction at viewing the results of my work, talking to my patients. I get to know them much better in these postoperative visits. We are old friends by now, I like them, they like me. It's very gratifying, and I can forget my troubles completely. I'm a little sorry when office hours are over. No more escape.

On our way up to Litchfield, Jim drives, as usual. Normally, I read. Today I stare out the window and think. Is there anything else I want to do with my life? No, I am doing exactly what I want, I love it, and I want to keep doing it. There is no unfinished business, nothing I wish I had done instead. My life is complete.

I am glad we had children when we were very young. At least they are nearly grown. I'm glad I changed careers, took the risk of going to medical school, found work that brings me joy. And I'm glad I found Jim so long ago, the epicenter of my life since I was seventeen. What will happen to Jim when I go? We have been so linked, almost fused, for so many years, I cannot fathom what this separation would be for him. It's unthinkable; maybe that's why he seems to have walled it off. I never thought I would die first, everyone knows women live longer than men, and he's older than I am. Look back, not forward.

I guess I'm very lucky. I have two wonderful children. Jim and I enjoy a happy relationship. I got the final sheepskin, board certification, last year. I am a partner in a first-rate orthopaedic group. I love my work, I'm very good at what I do. I have everything. Suddenly it hits me: the woman who has it all gets something more. I am overwhelmed with sadness.

SATURDAY, MAY 24, 1986

Today I have visits to make. I drive a quarter mile down the road to Reto's house. My brother, two years my junior, lives in Litchfield and works near Hartford, doing complex mathematical stuff on big computers for an insurance giant. He and Polly have three young boys, six, three, and one. I arrive amidst the usual morning swirl of children, cats, and a mutt big enough to pass for a pony.

Polly, Reto, and I settle down in the new, still incompletely finished, kitchen–family room, the children lose interest and wander off. I say I have to tell them something sad, and relate the news. They are very quiet. Reto looks at me and says, Well, I guess you get to create a miracle. Yeah, I say, without much conviction, I guess I do.

Polly asks, Is there anything, anything at all, we can do for you? No, nothing at all. The children don't know yet, but I think J will still want to spend the summer with them as planned as a mother's helper, as he did last summer. He very much wants to take driver's ed this summer so he can get his license as soon as possible after his birthday in August. He can do that up here, and he likes taking care of his cousins. If that's still what you want, I would like him to do that this summer, it would be better than his staying in New York, hanging around the apartment with nothing to do. Yes, of course we still want him. But there may be a problem with a bedroom, the construction hasn't gone as planned, and the woman who's been helping out here wants to stay longer than planned. J probably wouldn't mind staying in our house at night, he can walk or take his bike back and forth.

J's summer settled, bad news given, I depart, assuring them I'll keep them posted on progress, again repeat that this is a family secret, and though Mom knows and I'm going to tell Johnny and Joanie next, I'm holding off on Daddy and the children for now.

I turn down the road another half mile. My brother John is the youngest, nine years younger than I. John and Joan's children, four and one, look very much like our children. Though they live in the same apartment complex as we do in New York, they move to Litchfield for the summer and John commutes daily. They have just taken over the old colonial house where I grew up, halfway up the hill to my parent's new house, a large modern one finished in 1954.

I find John and Joan unpacking, getting organized. Strange to be in here, it seems much smaller than it did when I was nine or ten. We settle in the living room. The baby is being shy, clings to her mother. I tell the sad tale, it's getting easier with each telling. I finish, saying I'm determined to beat it. Joan says, with conviction, I know you will, Cesca, I just know you will—gosh, if anyone can beat it, it will be you. I tell her to hang on to those positive thoughts. John asks if I will need blood. No, not now, but maybe later I'll need platelets, it's better to get them from a single donor, but I don't need any now.

John asks, Have you contacted Lorraine? No, but I'm sure Mother has her on the case. John shrugs, half apologetically, at his inability to articulate what he's trying to say, finally says he is convinced it works, even if he can't say how or why, and cites his own example of recovering from acute abdominal pain that looked for all the world like a hot appendix. Don't knock it, John says. Right now, the way I see it, you need all the help you can get. Cautiously, I say, I'll see, but I am impressed that John, so oriented to the material world of Wall Street, can suspend his disbelief and gain value out of something so kooky as divine intervention called up on the phone from a spiritual teacher and healer.

I ask Joan not to tell her family, it's just for immediate family, no one else needs to know. And I'll tell them myself in my own time. It's really important to me to keep a lid on this, it's vital to my practice, I say. What I don't say is that I really don't want people talking about me, clucking sadly and sympathetically about this tragedy, which I feel, deep down, is my failure. And I don't want sympathy; sympathy could make me come unglued, right now I want to hold it together. The best way is to pretend to the world that nothing is happening. I can't face that special solace people extend to the dying. Then I'd have to be courageous, and I don't know how. Right now I feel scared and sad and very fragile.

I drive home. How'd it go? Jim asks. Fine, I say, now let's go find your parents. Jim's parents live in Litchfield, close to town, from May to October, and in Siesta Key, Florida, the rest of the time. His father, whose name is also Jim, retired as a general surgeon in 1973, the year I started medical school. He used to be chief of surgery at Roosevelt Hospital, and if it weren't for his influence, I might not be there now. He is a wonderful doctor, was the slickest surgeon around, nicknamed "the Jet," for his initials and for his dazzling speed on even the most difficult cases, not that he was slapdash, but because he was so good. Etty spent thirty-five years doing nearly full-time volunteer work at Roosevelt Hospital, too, and now spends all her time fussing over her husband. They are extremely devoted to each other and last year celebrated their fiftieth wedding anniversary.

The two Jims really are clones. Photographs of big Jim at thirty-eight are ringers for my Jim at the same age. I know what Jim will look like at eighty-two: he'll look seventy or younger, thin and slightly stoop-shouldered, hair still dark and thick, handsome forever. Big Jim has slowed down in recent years, medical problems have cut into his golf game and gardening, but he is still the kindest man in the world, still has a soft touch of genteel Texas in his manner and speech, always modest and unassuming, a gentle man. My Jim has often joked that I married him so I could talk to his father about medicine, my avid interest and vicarious pleasure in the years before I went to medical school myself.

Etty greets us outside, happy to see us; Jim is inside. We all move into the formal living room, big Jim and Etty on one sofa, Jim and me on its mate opposite. I tell the story again. Etty says with great sadness, Oh, Cesci, I feel I've just been kicked in the stomach. Big Jim is at a loss for words, no false cheer for him. We talk a bit about the chemo, Etty is solicitous. I ask them to keep this quiet.

Would you like to have dinner tonight or lunch tomorrow? Etty asks. Then you won't have to cook. No, thank you. Tonight we have a big cocktail party, and tomorrow we leave early for my secretary's wedding. Are you sure you feel up to it? Oh, yes, I want to go.

But, I say to Jim, I think I better get a hat, I have to stay out of the sun, and I need a big shady hat that will go with my dress. I also have in mind affecting hats now, a good way to cover my hair before it starts to look strange. Maybe no one will notice the difference under a hat, maybe I could even hide a wig, if it comes to that horrible eventuality. Jim laughs. Okay, we'll go look for a hat. He knows I love to shop in Litchfield, agrees to go along, even if it bores him. I need your advice, I say.

We go to The Workshop, a kind of kicky boutique. They have oodles of hats and I try on nearly every one. I settle on two straw numbers, they don't look too ridiculous, but I'm not sure I can pull this off, I'm really not a hat person. Jim says they look great. Jim affects boredom when I shop for clothes, but he has a good eye for what looks good on me, is emphatic about what he doesn't like and enthusiastic when he approves a selection. I have confidence in his opinions.

: :

SUNDAY, MAY 25, 1986

We leave for New York midmorning. It's a beautiful day for a wedding, hot and sunny. I have the directions, do the navigating to the middle reaches of Queens. We arrive at the church in plenty of time for the two o'clock wedding. We mill around with the people we know, all the secretaries at the office, meet their husbands and boyfriends. About quarter of, we go into the church, dark and cool. Jim and I are seated up close to the family pews, on the bride's side.

The wedding is on; Ruth is radiantly beautiful. I am caught up in the ceremony, Roman Catholic, but not so different from our Episcopalian one. I usually cry at weddings, this is no exception. I'm glad I remembered to stuff some Kleenex in my pocket. There are a whole bunch of prayers. I generally tune out on these, but all of a sudden, in the midst of some prayer for the blessing of children, long life, and grandchildren, I realize my loss. It is devastating. I will never see my grandchildren. I will never see Heather and J getting married. I might not even see them graduate from college. I will be gone so soon, too soon. These are bad thoughts, I must stop this, pull myself together.

Stay in the here and now. I focus instead on the priest, on his New York accent, on the way he pauses when a plane flies low and noisily overhead on its way to LaGuardia or Kennedy, much the way Keith Hernandez steps out of the batter's box and waits for the plane and the noise to pass over Shea before he gets set for a pitch.

After the ceremony, there is candid photography on the steps of the church. The bridal party departs for formal picture taking elsewhere. It is three in the afternoon, and the reception won't start till six. We all decide to go to a bar, where else? One of the men used to play guitar at a Spanish restaurant not too far away. We go there in convoy. We have fun, at least sixteen of us, listening to guitar strumming and singing along with old favorites, drinking. We have several rounds, I stick to orange juice. We almost hate to leave for the reception.

I'd been dreading this day, but the reception is a great party. Jim and I dance a bit, always enjoyable, but again we have to stop as I run out of breath and my legs and arms start to ache. We leave at eleven, and I have the sense the party may go all night. I know I can't go all night. I'm bushed, sleep in the car on the way home. Jim has an unerring sense of direction, can find his way home from anyplace.

MONDAY, MAY 26, 1986

We laze around the apartment all day, watch the baseball game on TV. I have a good idea about my hair: I'll get it colored to match the wig, then it won't be so noticeable if I have to switch to the wig. I'll do it tomorrow.

The phone rings. Hello, Cesca, It's Roopa—ah, Mimi. I

know, I recognize my younger sister's voice. She uses her Hindu name, Roopa, now, but the family still thinks of her by her family nickname of Mimi, and she habitually introduces herself by both names when she calls. Mother told me what's happening, she says. Oh, I was going to tell you, I'm sorry she did that. I feel a flare of anger. I told Mother it was a secret and I would tell my siblings myself, but I guess she had to talk to someone, and she and Mimi are on the same wavelength with their meditation groups and spiritual consciousness.

So how are you? Well, what can I say? It's pretty bad, a real shock—but my doctor is very positive that I can get into remission with this chemo. Good, good. I have you in my thoughts when I meditate, and it's very powerful to me, how strong you are, Cesca, like surrounded in a pure, white light. I know you are going to do well. This sounds kooky to me, but I say that's nice, keep it up, it might help, who knows? We talk some more about when she's coming East again, probably not till the end of the summer, and then hang up.

I call my mother and ask her not to tell my brother George or my sister Ginny, I'll do it myself when the time is right. George will be coming up for Ginny's daughter's wedding in June, and I don't want to burden Ginny with this now when she's so involved with both her children's weddings this summer. Let's wait and see what happens.

⋮

TUESDAY, MAY 27, 1986

⋮

An easy day today, just one short case and my clinic in the early afternoon. In the late afternoon I approach my hairdresser with my new wig in a bag. I explain that I want my hair colored to match it, leaving different shades, including some gray. Can you do that? Sure, no problem. My hair gets covered with some brown stuff, rinsed. There is a problem. This is red, I've never had red hair before, this is not the color we were talking about. He seems puzzled about how it turned out this way. He adds blue stuff, which tones it down, but the color is definitely auburn. I tell them I'm not happy, and I want it fixed some more. They say to come back tomorrow and we'll try again.

Jim doesn't like it either. Despite my anger, I recognize this is pretty funny: I get my hair colored to look like my wig so no one will notice, now I have a hair color everyone will notice, and it doesn't match the wig. Looks like I'm stuck with this color till my hair falls out, if it does.

WEDNESDAY, MAY 28, 1986

Today's surgery goes smoothly. I don't feel tired till I'm through in the early afternoon. No one mentions my new hair color, a sure sign it looks terrible: if you have nothing nice to say, say nothing.

The hairdresser, after multiple consultations with the other colorists, "drabs" the color. A miniscule difference. I note that my hair color is easier to worry about than the myeloma, the fatigue.

THURSDAY, MAY 29, 1986

I rush to make my appointment with Anne before my office hours start. First my bloods are drawn, a CBC and also a viscosity, which is a measure of the effect of the elevated protein caused by the myeloma. The viscosity was high last week, just keeping an eye on it. Anne checks my blood pressure, lungs, and eyeballs again. Everything still normal, very good.

What do I tell the kids, Anne? I don't know how to explain it. I start to cry again. Anne is sympathetic, yet practical. You have to tell them the truth, Cesca, they are intelligent, and they have access to your books too. They will be able to read about it. You should use the words *cancer* and *chemotherapy,* but just don't use any numbers or dates for prognosis, that won't help them. And make sure they don't get it confused with melanoma, many people do because the words sound so similar. Yes, I think, and the prognosis for melanoma can be worse than my disease.

I dash home after office hours to change for dinner at a fancy new fish restaurant with friends from out of town. Anne calls me at home, reaches me just as I'm about to leave. My bloods came back, my hematocrit is down a bit, to 23, but that's all right. However, the viscosity is elevated, up to 7.5 from 5, normal is less than 2. None of this means much to me; I don't know anything about serum viscosity.

Anne goes on, I think we need to do something soon to lower the viscosity. Like what? Plasmapheresis, it's like dialysis, they can reduce the level of protein in your serum immediately, so we don't have to wait for the chemo to kick in and do it. What's the rush? Well, we don't want anything bad to happen, something we can prevent. What could happen? Well, you could have a stroke. Oh, no. I suddenly realize Anne is telling me I could die right now. I might die before the weekend, before Heather graduates, before I tell the children I'm sick. I'm a time bomb with a short fuse. Or, worse, I could become a vegetable.

Do we do it tonight? No, I think tomorrow is soon enough. Where? I've talked to the guy in charge and he's going to call you at your office tomorrow morning about eight and set it up with you. Is it okay to wait? Yes, I think so. Just drink a lot of fluids, really force it. Don't worry, I will.

I drink two big glasses of water before I leave. I'm in shock, can't believe death is this close. No, it can't be so. Jim's on his way to the restaurant where we're meeting our friends, can't reach him.

Dinner is delicious, I suppose. Mostly I drink water and shuttle to the ladies' room. I listen to the table talk with half an ear, realize I'm distracted, try to look like I'm present.

On the way home in the cab, I explain the latest development to Jim, downplay it for my benefit. Go to sleep and hope I wake up. Actually, I wake up often to go to the bathroom, drink more water all night long. No wonder I've been so thirsty for so long, I've been compensating for this elevated protein, the high viscosity.

FRIDAY, MAY 30, 1986

After my session with the residents and rounds on my patients, I go across the street to the office. I call the plasmapheresis guy, who was a resident when I was an intern. He expresses sympathy, emphasizes that Anne has explained the confidentiality issue, and assures me he'll keep it quiet. He offers me an appointment in his research lab at the Rogosin Kidney Center at noon. Fine, I say, that'll be perfect, my office hours will be over by then.

Are these the renal dialysis machines, can I get hepatitis from this? No, these are different, we use new tubing on each patient, spin the blood down in a centrifuge, give you back your cells with albumin, throw out your own serum, no chance of any contact with anybody else's blood, no risk at all, you'll see. Can I drive myself home after this, will I be faint or woozy? No, you can drive.

I meet him in the small research lab. There are two machines, one on each side of the room. A lounge chair is next to each one. Someone else is across from me, looks vaguely familiar. I pay attention to the nurse, who hooks up a very large needle to each elbow vein, straps my arms out straight on two boards. Now I'm really helpless, can't use either arm. How long is this going to take? About two hours. The nurse puts a pillow in my lap, arranges the newspaper so I can read it. We'll turn the pages for you, don't you try to do it.

Blood flows out my right arm, gets spun down in the machine next to me, out of my line of sight, the plasma is siphoned off, the red cells, white cells, and platelets are remixed with packaged albumin, and the less viscous mix flows in to my left arm. This one treatment can knock my protein level down as much as forty percent, which should get my viscosity into a safer range. The plasmapheresis guy explains that viscosity is weird, there's a certain level at which even a small increase just stops blood flow in small vessels. Like my brain, I think. What level of viscosity? About 8. Mine is 7.5, and rising from last week. I'm relieved to be here, grateful to Anne for anticipating the problem.

The man in the chair opposite looks me in the eye. Dr. Thompson, how nice to see you. Oh, no. One of my patients, of all people! He is here getting his one hundred and first plasmapheresis, he announces proudly. He has a peripheral neuropathy caused by some unknown circulating antibody, and washing it out of his blood controls the nerve damage, enables him to continue to walk, take care of himself.

I explain to him that I am here for an illness that I want no one, especially other patients and his doctor, to know about, and I ask him to pretend he has not seen me. He assures me that before he became a professor, he was a rabbi, and my secret is safe with him, it's like a priest in your confessional, wild horses could not drag it out of him. I thank him, and we chat about what he's been doing for the last couple of years for a few minutes until I can escape into my newspaper.

This isn't so bad, I think. Just wash out the high protein that can gum up my works. If, when, the chemo can no longer control the plasma cells, maybe I'll be able to buy more time with this plasmapheresis. Very controllable, amazing what can be done nowadays. And this doesn't make you sick like renal dialysis. I feel quite relieved and comforted. I wouldn't like giving up several hours a week to this, but, all in all, not a bad trade-off to control this disease.

I have to go the john, badly. How much longer is this going to take? I ask. About another half hour, forty-five minutes. I don't think I can wait that long, but I try. I've been forcing fluids all morning, and now I'm getting a large amount of albumin and saline, probably more than is being removed. After twenty minutes I tell the nurse she has to unhook me so I can go to the ladies' room. Not necessary, she says. She surrounds my chair with a screen for privacy, brings in a bedpan, helps me onto it. This isn't very private, but I'm too desperate to care. The bedpan is too small, overflows, and I am unable to stop. I remember, guiltily, being a kid in a swimming pool, having too much fun to leave the pool to pee.

Soon the plasmapheresis is over, two hours and twenty minutes. The plasmapheresis guy returns, says I'll probably feel much better after this treatment, and I should have another one early next week. How's Tuesday afternoon? Fine.

Before leaving, I call Anne, tell her it went well. She tells me to take it easy this weekend, stay out of the sun. I remind her that it's Heather's graduation, that may be impossible. Wear a big hat then, and take water with you, drink a lot. Okay.

Jim and I drive up to Litchfield, have just enough time to change for the parents' dinner at Taft. I take my camera, photograph Heather and her friends. It is stifling in the gym, my hair is soaked. Heather is intrigued by the new color, I tell her I got tired of the gray. We leave as soon as possible, around nine. Heather is very happy, this is a real milestone in her life.

SATURDAY, MAY 31, 1986

Jim and I have breakfast on the deck. It's a beautiful summery morning, the air is lush and dewy. We talk about Heather's big day, what we can give her for graduation that will really mean something to her. She knows we are planning to buy her a hi-fi set, when she decides what kind she wants. This doesn't seem momentous enough to me. I suggest to Jim that she is an adult now, will be eighteen soon and has earned adult privileges. He agrees readily, I'm actually the one who has been reluctant to let her go.

I write Heather a letter. I feel acutely that I need to give her something that will convince her she has truly done well in our eyes, my eyes, something that will set herself to rest when I die and am no longer there for her. I want her to have a sense of my love and approval to keep with her for all time.

I write. I congratulate her, tell her we are very proud of her achievements and love her very much. That when we love our children, we want to protect them from bad things that can happen, but this is not always possible as they get older. That she has demonstrated that she can take responsibility for herself and she has earned that privilege. That henceforth she can go where she wants, when she wants. She can drive with anyone she chooses. She can have anyone visit the apartment or house when we are not there. She can stay out as late as she wants. She is on her own. This is her graduation present from us.

We arrive early for the graduation exercises, stake out choice seats for the large family contingent. All the seats are in full sun. I stash a small ice chest with water and a bottle of champagne under a seat, carry my camera. Heather is more gorgeous than usual, surrounded by several friends, all boys, naturally, who have traveled hundreds of miles all night to share this occasion with her. I give her the letter I wrote, she stuffs it in her pocket, distracted by her friends. I'm a little disappointed that she doesn't read it immediately. She leaves to change into her graduation robes.

Speeches, prizes, handing out of diplomas. Heather is radiant, triumphant. Her grandparents and godparents, my brother Reto and Jim's sister Betsy, are there to shower her with presents as well. Heather thanks us for our letter too. The relatives depart, Heather's friends stay, and we walk slowly to an outdoor picnic for family and friends. Heather notices my limp, asks if I'm okay. Just a little back and leg pain, I've had this before. You go on, I'll catch up in a little while.

We sit under a shady tree for our picnic. I give the chilled champagne to Heather and her friends, take pictures of the group. After the picnic Jim goes to get the car so I won't have to walk the quarter mile. Heather accompanies me to the road, asks again if I'm really okay. Yes, I'm fine, just a little backache. Why is it I don't believe you? she asks darkly. I think to myself, Because you've always been intuitive and sensitive, that's why you have so many friends who love you, but I say only, I'll get over it soon, it's just annoying.

Heather asks if a friend can stay with us in New York for a couple of days before she returns home. Sure, I say, somewhat dismayed that I'll have to postpone telling Heather the truth about my illness, yet relieved as well to postpone this most difficult of all the tellings.

We spend the afternoon emptying Heather's room into a borrowed pickup truck to cart home. Jim and J and Heather do all the grunt work, I observe and drive the delicate framed pictures and computer equipment in the car. Heather leaves to go to the big graduation blast someplace in Fairfield County. I urge her to spend the night at the party rather than drive anywhere with anyone who's been drinking, unable to resist this admonition despite the new manifesto. Heather agrees, says she's planning to take the train in to New York Sunday afternoon, will see us there. J stays at school; he has exams this week, won't get out till next weekend.

Jim and I go to his parents' for supper. Jim's sister, Betsy, is staying there. I take her for a walk down the road, tell her the story. What can I do for you to help? Nothing, really, except be available for Heather and J, they may need to talk to someone else about this as time goes on. We walk back uphill and I notice that I'm not so out of breath, my calves don't ache. Things are getting better, I think, the plasmapheresis really helped. Yes, we really can control this disease, just like diabetes or hypertension. No sweat.

SUNDAY, JUNE 1, 1986

After breakfast I go look for my father at my parents' house. He's not at home, so I drive to the farm, a quarter mile down the road, where he spends most of his time in his workshop, fixing up old cars, inventing gadgets. Daddy has become reclusive in recent years, eats and sleeps and works on his own time schedule, quite unpredictable, refuses to go out socially, even to family gatherings. He also doesn't trim his beard or cut his hair very often; with his beetle brows he bears a striking resemblance to the Ayatollah Khomeini. We think a large part of this eccentricity is due to his refusal to use a hearing aid, but he is adamant in his assertion that he is old enough to do just what he wants, and what he wants is to be left alone, accompanied by his adoring companion, a tiny Yorkshire terrier.

Itsy-Bitsy greets me with bounces and barks, heralds my arrival. Daddy is delighted to see me, invites me in, turns down the volume of the classical music on the radio. We sit down to chat, I shout so he'll hear me. Daddy, I have something very sad to tell you. Oh, no, what is it? I am sick, I have a bone marrow cancer. Cancer? You? What does this mean? Well, with chemotherapy I may live quite a while, but it's not curable. He starts to cry, and so do I.

Oh, Tati, he says, reverting to my childhood name, I wish it were me and not you, why can't it be me? Because life isn't fair, Daddy. The distance that has built up between us in the past years of his retreat from the world is instantly dissolved. His love for me is manifest directly; he would die for me if he could. I know I was always his favorite child, he took great pride in my achievements. I disappointed him greatly when I did not change my name back to Morosani on my graduation from medical school. It would have pleased him enormously to have a Dr. Morosani among his children, a real achievement for an immigrant who never finished high school. That doesn't matter anymore. He would die so I could live. And I would accept that sacrifice, if it were possible.

I can give you my blood, we have the same type. I look at him, frail and wizened, and say, No, Daddy, you need your blood, and anyway, I don't need it now. We talk some more. I swear him to secrecy, not really necessary

76

because he doesn't communicate with many people. I assure him I'll keep him up to date on my progress.

Mother comes over in the afternoon while we're watching the Mets game. I'm more hooked on baseball than ever, can lose myself in the game totally. She gives me a book, urges me to read it. *The Art of Spiritual Healing*, by Joel Goldsmith. Oh, no, I think, here we go. Mother says she's been talking to Lorraine, gives me her address and phone number so I can call and write myself. Okay, I assent, I guess it can't hurt.

Later, in the car on the way to New York, I start the book. Heavy going, stilted biblical language. I persevere through a chapter or two, it doesn't make much sense to me.

TUESDAY, JUNE 3, 1986

My work is my sanctuary. Time flies, I don't have to think about my disease, I enjoy what I am doing, transcend everything in the flow of the moment. I am lucky to have this.

My second plasmapheresis goes smoothly. The thirtyish man opposite me is a research patient on a new protocol developed to demonstrate whether plasmapheresis can alter the life expectancy of people with abnormally high lipids in the blood, cholesterol levels in the 500s, rather than the normal 200. People with such high lipid levels are doomed to early death from heart disease. This is an interesting application of a new technology. The guy across from me is optimistic, feels grateful to be part of something that may make a difference for him. I envy him, wish there were something for me too.

I check in with Anne again before I leave. No need to set up another treatment, we'll see what my viscosity and CBC are from the bloods drawn today, and I'll go see her on Friday this week. Yes, I'm feeling fine, maybe even better.

WEDNESDAY, JUNE 4, 1986

After an easy day of office hours, I return home. This I dread. Heather's friend has left, and I've run out of excuses. Heather has to be told. She has a summer job selling coffee beans in a tourist shop in the South Street Seaport and comes home in the evening, after we've had dinner. I sit down with her on the sofa in the living room, tell her I have more to tell her about my anemia, that further tests are back. I have too many plasma cells in my marrow, it's a form of bone marrow cancer called multiple myeloma, and that's why I got anemic. I have started chemotherapy, which should control it very well for a long time.

Heather sobs, throws herself in my lap: Don't leave me now, I've just gotten you back! We hug each other. I know what she means. We had been at loggerheads for some time, mutual resentments piled up for an explosion last Christmas vacation, which cleared the air. Heather had been sullen about the rules of the house, the curfew, all the restrictions imposed by her unrelenting parents.

This was fueled, I knew, by her deep resentment of what she viewed as my abandonment of her during the years of my medical training. I leveled with her then, told her that I wasn't just working for my personal fulfillment, as great as it is, but that as a family we knew way back then that we would need my income to educate her and J in the way they were now being educated. Sacrifices had to be made, and hers was to be deprived of my presence more than she liked. It had been hard for her, I knew, but it was unavoidable.

But I like you when you are my friend, not my mother. Yes, I like that, too, but I am your mother first, you are still in high school, and it is my responsibility to protect you now, whether you like it or not.

Our relationship lightened up considerably after that confrontation. Over spring vacation we became even closer as I began to realize that Heather was the same age I was when Jim and I began our relationship, that it was possible that her attachment to her boyfriend was serious and adult, that she was, in fact, as adult as I was at the same age. No wonder she felt she had just gotten me back. We had laid to rest the years-long mother-daughter conflict. I was glad we got through that before this illness came along.

I tell her that I was sorry to have held this news back, but I hadn't wanted to spoil her graduation. I would keep her up to date on my treatment, and she could ask me about it anytime. I explain to her about the plasmapheresis, emphasizing the opportunities to control this disease with modern medical technology.

FRIDAY, JUNE 6, 1986

A long weekend. We are on our summer schedule because Jim's office rearranges the work schedule so everyone works longer every day and has every other Friday off. I can easily accommodate my schedule to that as well.

After my teaching session with the residents and rounds on my patients at Roosevelt Hospital, I drive over to Anne's office at New York Hospital and park in the garage across the street.

First the blood-drawing, then Anne checks me over. Everything still looks fine, I'm doing well, Anne assures me. My white blood cell count should be down to a little below normal because of the chemo, but it will go lower next week, and we should check it again then. Yes, I remember, the "nadir" of the counts, that day or so when the white blood cell count hits its lowest point before the cells recover from the effect of the chemo and start growing again.

Chemotherapy attacks rapidly dividing cells, and the effects on the white blood cells necessary for defense against infection are evidenced about two weeks after the dose is given. We need to see how low the white cells get to gauge whether the current dose is too much. The idea is to give enough to have an effect on the malignant plasma cells without totally wiping out the white cells I need. As long as my white count stays above 1, for a thousand white cells per milliliter of blood, I'm in the safe range, although 2 is better.

We agree to meet again on June 10, Tuesday. I will be giving a talk on foot problems at the Update Your Medicine course at Cornell that afternoon and will also pick up my slides for the talk I'm giving in Vail in July, so I'll be able to get a lot done on one trip across town. Anne says she'll call me with the results of today's test later. No, I better call you, we're going up to Litchfield, so you'd have a hard time reaching me.

Anne reminds me that she wants me to take it easy, not work too hard. I say that I've been thinking of taking every Friday off this summer, that won't be too noticeable and will give me a long rest on the weekends. Good, Cesca, do that.

We pick J up at school, cart some of his stuff home, and then Jim and J return for the rest of it with our old Volvo station wagon. While they're gone, I check in with Anne. White count down to 2.4 from 9, a very good response, not too much, not too little, 4 to 11 is considered normal range, so I'm low, as expected, but not dangerously so.

After J has unloaded his stuff—computer, overstuffed chair, hi-fi—Jim and I sit with him in the living room. I tell him about my illness, a family secret, choosing my words carefully, likening this disease to other chronic diseases like hypertension and diabetes, but still use the words *cancer, chemotherapy, plasmapheresis.* J is phlegmatic, intrigued by the elevated protein, asks questions about the technique of plasmapheresis. He has learned some details of protein synthesis in biology this year, tries to fit this into that framework. We discuss it a bit, and then he wanders off.

No impact, it didn't register. Jim looks at me, says, Gee, it's too bad about that hangnail you have. I don't know if Jim is referring to how I just underplayed the reality or how J reacted. I wonder if I said it wrong, decide that J will come to an understanding of this later, when he's ready to absorb it, but I feel vaguely guilty about how

I put it out there. I realize that for a moment I believed that this was a trivial medical problem, of no real consequence, really, and J picked up that conviction.

WEEKEND, JUNE 7 AND 8, 1986

We have a festive time. Karen and Cox arrive after lunch, Bill and Linda in time for dinner. Everyone but Linda knows about my illness, nobody discusses it except for quiet questions about how I'm feeling when they can get me aside. I'm fine, I say, better than I was, in fact. I very much enjoy being with friends, relaxing, sharing a good meal and the great wine Bill brought along. I have a glass. This is normalcy, I want to maintain my normal life, and damn it, I will.

TUESDAY, JUNE 10, 1986

I practice my talk in the morning before I operate. I've given this one several times, it's a matter of anticipating which slide is next so my transitions will be smooth. I am ready, very much want this talk to go well, it's the first time I've given a talk in the main auditorium at my own medical school to an audience of internists and general practitioners.

Before the talk, I go to Anne's lab for the blood drawing, set up an appointment for Friday morning. My suit covers the telltale Band-Aid at my elbow. I look healthy, I decide, no one could guess I'm on chemotherapy, at the nadir of my counts. I feel like I'm living a double life.

My presentation is about the ten most common foot and ankle problems I see, and solutions to them, both operative and conservative. It goes over very well, there are many interested questions at the end, and it takes me a while to extricate myself from the stragglers.

Before going home I pick up my slides at the photography department at the Hospital for Special Surgery and take the time to look up some friends there I haven't seen for a while. I always enjoy seeing them, but more important, I want them to see me looking healthy and vigorous, just in case any rumors surface about my illness; they would not believe it, having just seen me looking great and obviously active.

FRIDAY, JUNE 13, 1986

No office hours today. I see Anne for more blood tests and a checkup. All is well, as usual. Can we cut down to once-a-week blood tests? I ask. Yes, that will be okay. Your counts should be coming up again next week, but we need to confirm it so we can plan the next round of chemo, five weeks after the first.

I report that I'm feeling so much better that I've resumed the cross-country ski machine, am up to two whatevers, miles or kilometers, which takes me about ten or twelve minutes. The back pain has improved with Feldene, which I'm tolerating well, and the stretching exercises, boring but effective. Soon I plan to start walking, maybe, because I read that myeloma patients who walk a lot do better.

Anne is enthusiastic in her agreement, says walking has been a cardinal principle in myeloma treatment for years, but she also admonishes me not to consider running, that would not be advisable, please don't get carried away. I think of the envy with which I regard the runners I see in the park, feeling about a hundred years old and crippled as I drive by, and say, wryly, There's little chance I'll ever be able to do that again.

Anne tells me she's going on vacation for a few weeks and has arranged for another hematologist in her office to take over for her with me while she's away, and he is very discreet, won't breathe a word. I remember him, we were interns the same year, he in medicine and me in surgery, but I worked with him closely on one of my medical rotations. He was a good doc then, and I'm sure he is now. Even so, I feel a pang that Anne will be far away if I need her. I remind myself that all doctors need to get totally away at least once, preferably twice, a year in order to have fun at work. If it works that way for me, it must be doubly true for an oncologist.

I tell Anne that I hate bothering her about the blood tests, and I know the secretaries are not allowed to report blood results to patients over the phone. I've tried calling the lab, but they just have inpatient results coded in. Anne smiles, says, I may as well tell you because I know you, Cesca, you'll figure it out on your own. Just use 1 as a prefix to your hospital ID number, and they'll have what they need to code in. We agree that she'll call me if she has any concerns over the results, I'll call her if I have any questions, but otherwise I can just get my results direct from the lab. I feel gratified by this solution, much more in control of what's going on with me. She tells me not to worry if the CBC isn't in the computer the same day, they run those tests in their own lab, and a day later they get entered in the computer bank.

The new system works. In the afternoon I learn from the lab that my viscosity is 2.1, nearly normal, definitely not dangerous, no need for more plasmapheresis. And the total protein is down to 9, a big step from the 18 it was two weeks ago. Definite progress, but probably more the effect of the plasmapheresis than the chemo at this point. But this is certainly proving to be a controllable disease.

I settle into my usual routine: get up early, exercise, buff up my talk for the Vail meeting, go to the office or operate. Pick up dinner at the gourmet take-out, watch the baseball game with Jim. His excitement and enthusiasm parallels mine. He was a rabid Yankee fan in childhood and he played with friends into his teens. Now he relishes my attention to the Mets, the stats, and various players' foibles. This is another way we can enjoy our time together. J, up in the country at his baby-sitting job, often calls us during a game to crow about an especially spectacular play. Heather's at home but frequently out with friends at night, working in the coffee store downtown. Thank goodness she doesn't feel she has to hover.

At work Bill, Fiske, and Drew act normal with me, treat me the same as ever, are interested in my progress but gratifyingly unsolicitous in their concern. They make it easy for me to talk to them, no treading on eggshells. I report with pleasure that I have noted the insidious onset of wellness, am surprised that I hadn't noticed how dragged-out I had been. Denial is a funny thing, recognizable only in retrospect.

I start thinking about my will. We both need new wills,

have needed them since the law changed last year, but never got around to it. Now we really have to do something. My partner Charlie has a father in an established firm that handles this kind of thing. I ask Charlie to ask his father if there is some young person at the firm who could help us out with this. Charlie hooks us up right away, we set up an appointment for June 18. I press for getting this done as soon as possible. We're both flying together on a trip to Vail soon and shouldn't leave this unfinished, God forbid something should happen. I'm just superstitious, I add apologetically.

Before we go to the meeting with the lawyers, Jim asks if I'm going to level with them about my illness. No way. There's no need for them to know; the whole point of a will is to handle things when you die, they don't need to know I might die soon. I'm relieved that I kept the secret as we have our initial meeting, because one of the lawyers turns out to have a son starting at J's school and her husband is an internist who refers patients to me. Small world. Not that secrets aren't kept by lawyers, but still it's too close for me.

In my spare time I struggle with some of Mother's books. *The Art of Spiritual Healing* is going slowly. My brother John advises me to hang in there with it; even if it doesn't make much sense to my rational mind, I might absorb it by osmosis.

There are more books from my mother. She expresses her love by deluging me with books of inspiration and example. One of them captures my imagination: *Why Me?* by a young boy who miraculously recovered from a malignant, inoperable brain tumor, details an approach newly designated psychoneuroimmunology. By combining relaxing techniques, a form of self-hypnosis, this boy spent a good deal of time every day imagining his white cells attacking his tumor, gobbling it up like a bunch of Pac-Men at war. After some months of this, and good old-fashioned radiation therapy, he went searching in his imagination for some spongy old tumor cells for his white cells to munch on and found nothing but a small, glistening white scar. He reported to his psychologist-guide in this experiment that the tumor was gone. Soon after, a follow-up CAT scan confirmed his imagined observation: no more tumor, just dense tissue where the tumor had been. The book was written some years after his expected demise, and he had remained tumor free. He still spent time setting his white cells on alert for invaders.

My rational mind says this is an anecdote. "Anecdotal" is a medical scientist's perjorative designation used in rebuttal of the validity of an isolated occurrence. He may believe he recovered because he engaged his imagination to marshal his immune system to destroy his tumor selectively, but that does not prove it happened that way. Maybe he was just lucky. Maybe the radiation was effective in this instance. Still . . . it's intriguing.

I find myself roaming through my bone marrow while dreamy in the early morning, half awake, not wanting to start the day so early. I see countless purple-blue spheres, my myeloma cells; I look around for some helpers, some troops I can call in, white knights. What do those natural killer cells look like? The task seems hopeless, so many blue balls. I marshal my forces, instruct them to go on autopilot, pop those blue babies until they hear from me again. I slip back into sleep. My rational mind tells me this is stupid, but I tell myself it beats crying, something I seem to do quite often in the quiet of near sleep.

FRIDAY, JUNE 20, 1986

I see Anne's substitute today. We reminisce about the internship year we shared. He asks how I'm feeling. Now that you mention it, I feel like a truck hit me since I came off the prednisone, it's some withdrawal. No wonder it's hard to get people off the stuff when they're taking it for asthma or arthritis. Do you have musculoskeletal pain? No, just fatigue. He tells me about his experience with prednisone, which he had to take in high dose for an acoustic neuroma. During withdrawal he hurt all over, every tendon and muscle in his body felt inflamed. Very unpleasant, he commiserates, but you should feel better soon.

I ask him about the acoustic neuroma. He admits it was very scary before it was diagnosed, still scary because he's going to have it removed with some very delicate brain surgery later this summer. A benign tumor, but malignant in its growth, taking up brain space behind the ear. Yes, he'll have permanent hearing loss in that ear. We both know the scariest part is getting through the surgery without brain damage. We doctors are partial to our brainpower. I feel I am talking to a kindred soul; he knows where I'm at, he is there, too.

We arrange the chemo for Thursday next week, if my counts look okay today. All the same, I should come in the day before and get another CBC just to be safe. I leave him and wait for my blood work to be drawn, no rush because I'm not working today.

SATURDAY, JUNE 21, 1986

I check with the lab on Saturday. White count 4.7, normal; hematocrit up to 29 from a low of 23. Good, the chemo must be working, my marrow's making red cells for me. Viscosity stable at 2.2.

Looks like I'll be able to go with the next round of chemo next week. I calculate whether the chemo will interfere with what I want to do. I won't take the zombie medicine, Compazine, this time. If I'm sick the day after, that's okay, it's Friday and I won't be in the office. If my white count drops it should be up again before my trip to Vail, that's good.

Next weekend we'll be on Long Island for my niece's wedding. I'll see my brother George there and tell him then. It should be a fun weekend, the whole family will be staying at a conference center, a resort spa.

Our weekends have become very sedate. I don't feel like doing anything except sitting on the deck in the shade and reading. Last summer we biked about six miles a day, spent a lot of time clearing brush and trees, real lumberjack work. It's out of the question for me. Jim doesn't mind, is content to sit with me on the deck reading; we have always been in synchronous, almost symbiotic, orbit with each other in our nonworking time, following individual proclivities together, whether hiking trails, cooking for dinner parties, skiing, whatever. Neither of us has been inclined to go off and pursue activities alone, our focus has always been to be with each other.

We see J on the weekends, he's living in our house and working for Reto and Polly, seems to be having an okay time. We have dinner with my family, rotating houses, contributing various courses: you do the main course, I'll do the salad, so-and-so will do dessert, very informal, very last minute.

I think vaguely about entertaining; we owe a lot of people. I don't feel up to it, not just the work, but the planning seems too much to think about. Besides, I would rather avoid the people I know, not just acquaintances, but friends too. Pretending that things are okay when our life has crashed down around us is too hard. I have noticed that I answer obliquely when people ask how I am: the kids are fine, Jim is great, my practice is going well, I'm very busy. Very satisfactory answers, very much off the mark.

THURSDAY, JUNE 26, 1986

Chemo, round two. Same IV dose of Cytoxan, vincristine, BCNU. One week of Alkeran, one week of prednisone at high dose, 60 milligrams, then taper to none over the next week. Anne's substitute tells me Anne likes a fast taper, next time it might even be faster. Good. The less the better, from my point of view. Maybe it won't hit me so hard coming off if I'm not on it as long.

I tell him I haven't noticed any hair loss yet, does he think it might happen this time? Hard to say, probably not. How long do you think I'll have to stay on this regimen? He says he likes to keep his patients on it for eighteen months. Even if they're in remission before then? I think my hair will never last that long.

Well, he says, nobody really knows much about this. Used to be people were on daily Alkeran and prednisone in low dose forever. Now with the M2 protocol people get into remission sooner, but it's not really established as to how long is enough before going off it entirely. He thinks Anne may lean toward less time, maybe a year. I don't like this uncertainty. I remember that Anne had said it was controversial.

I reflect on my avoidance of looking at the literature

on myeloma treatment. I had discussed this with Drew, who told me he knew nothing about it and wasn't going to look, wanted to wall off the area. I had the sense he felt no news was good news, what he didn't know wouldn't bother him. He was satisfied to hear from me about it.

I told him that I sensed that whatever I would find in the literature would already be out of date, that I was relying on Anne to interpret the data she heard at meetings, where the hot new stuff is reported. Even more important is what people discuss informally at these meetings at coffee breaks and meals, that's where the real communication occurs. So much is cleaned up and truncated in scientific reports. You have to know who is reporting data, what their bias is, are they reliable? Even in science, especially clinical science, much has to be taken with a barrel of salt. I don't have the background to interpret the literature in context. Anne will have to do that for me. But maybe it wouldn't hurt to take a little peek in the library.

WEEKEND, JUNE 27–29, 1986

Tori's wedding weekend, hot, clear summer weather. We settle in at the conference center in the late afternoon, rendezvous with my family, whose rooms are near ours. George won't be there till tomorrow. The rehearsal dinner is fun, much toasting.

The wedding is lovely. Having gotten through Ruth's wedding, this one is not hard for me at all. The reception is at Piping Rock. About halfway through the reception, I ask my brother George to come take a walk with me so we can talk. We stroll across the lawns looking out over the acres of golf course. Bad news, George. I tell him the story. He puts his arm around me and we keep walking, talking. I emphasize the positive, but he is in tears, he is not fooled. He offers me blood, anything. I say we may need to check his tissue type, see if we match. Anytime. And don't tell your children.

EARLY JULY, 1986

I'm busy at work, I work on my Vail talk, organize my slides. My energy is improving all the time, the shortness of breath has disappeared. Did I really have it? In idle moments I project to the future, which has become an amorphous gray zone of time. Things are going all right, this thing is under control. I still have hair, I'm not sick.

I think about the more radical treatment Anne alluded to—harvesting bone marrow to freeze for "later." I picture a team of surgeons operating on my bones, reaming out the long bones and saving the marrow. Would I have to be on crutches? Would I even be able to use crutches? Would I be stuck in bed waiting for my bones to heal? I have no substantive framework to drape my fantasies on. What's the point of saving marrow if it still has some tumor cells in it? It only takes one bad cell to carry on the disease, right?

This sounds too dangerous. Not only that, I'd have to stop working.

I talk to Fiske. I want to maximize my chances of a long survival, but I don't want to compromise what I can do now. I want to keep working, get the kids educated, four more years for Heather, seven for J, not counting graduate school; I guess that's my first responsibility. Don't rock the boat, keep going. Fiske is a good listener, allows me to focus my conflicting thoughts, doesn't tell me what to do. It is such a relief to have friends to talk to. I tend to go in circles on my own, get bogged down in despair. As the song goes, I get by with a little help from my friends. How true.

On my way to Liver Rounds, a beer party for the residents on the roof of the hospital, I stop at the Roosevelt Hospital library to see what I can find on multiple myeloma. My curiosity has overcome my reluctance to investigate on my own, my previous resolve to let Anne be my interpreter.

I find the *Index Medicus* on the counter, look over listings on multiple myeloma. Not that many. I skip over impenetrable titles about kinetics, or drugs I've never heard of, or mice experiments; no way I'll make sense of those. Here's a good one: "Multiple Myeloma: A Review of 869 Cases," by Dr. Kyle at the Mayo Clinic. The first sentence makes the hairs on the back of my neck stand up: "Ten-year survival with multiple myeloma is remarkable." Hey, wait a second, I thought this was indolent and took a long time. I have a heavy, sinking feeling as I read on, scan the graphs. Median survival is twenty months—that's less than two years for half the people. I'm in tears now, surreptitiously looking around to see if anyone can see me. Good, the library is empty. Only ten percent survive five years. Shit. Of the few ten-year survivors, half died within two years of leukemia caused by long-term use of alkylating drugs. Alkeran, Cytoxan—both alkylating drugs. Great. If the tumor don't get you, the treatment will. I have to talk to Anne about this. This was written in 1975, long before the M2 protocol. But, even if survival is longer, I sense the principle will be the same: long-term chemo creates new leukemias that will kill you. My chances of beating these odds seem very slim—and what a way to live, waiting for the other shoe to drop.

I put the book away, pull myself together, go up to the roof and have a couple of beers with the residents and some other attendings. A little beer is okay, the anti-ulcer medicine, Zantac, is protecting me. I'll think about the future tomorrow, for now I'll just keep going as if nothing were different. Shut it out, live in the moment. I envy Jim's ability to do that, but I'm getting better at it.

JULY 7, 1986

Anne's finally back from her vacation. I meet with her first thing Monday morning. Bloods drawn, listen to lungs, check eyes. All is well. We sit down to talk. I tell her what I read about the Mayo experience. Suddenly the intellectual mask slips, my rage and frustration surface, and I say fiercely, Anne, I want to beat this fucker.

Momentarily stunned by my vehemence, Anne recovers quickly, says, Of course, you do. So do I. You are so young, so healthy, we should try something radical.

I'll do anything, I say, whatever it takes, I just want to beat it. Now. What's out there? I don't really know, Anne says, I'll have to talk to people, find out who's doing something innovative. I know they're not doing anything besides M2 at Memorial. In the meantime, in case we want to do a transplant, we should set up tissue typing for your family, find out if you have a match with any of your brothers and sisters. You have a bunch, right? Four full siblings, one half sister, she wouldn't count. Your parents ought to be matched, too; it helps them to sort out the next generation.

The whole family will be coming through New York for the next family wedding at the end of August, that would be the best time, but I know they would all come at the drop of a hat if we need to do it sooner.

No, that should be plenty of time. Try to remember, Cesca, you are doing very, very well. She smiles, pleased with our results so far. Your immunoelectrophoresis from two weeks ago is back, the IgG level is down to 3600 from 11,000, that's very, very good. Yeah, but a lot of that is the plasmapheresis, which is just temporary. Some, but not all of it. I think you are responding very well to the chemo, which is good news.

I'm going to Vail next week for the Foot and Ankle Society meeting, to give a talk, and play. Jim's coming with me to look after me. Anne looks thoughtful, says, I think that will be okay, just be sure to get a lot of rest. That's no problem, the meetings are only in the morning, and I won't do anything strenuous in the afternoon.

THURSDAY, JULY 17, 1986

I have too much time to think on the plane to Vail. We signed the wills before we left, so my "affairs are in order"—what a strange expression! Some of my partners have often joked that we are so heavily insured in our Keogh plan that we're worth more dead than alive. That's not really true, but I calculate that the interest alone from my insurance benefits will cover the upcoming education expenses for Heather and J, and if Jim and my brothers as executors manage the estate well, there should be a cushion for Jim, too, with considerable belt tightening.

So I can gamble with my life a bit, take a chance that might not work out. I can put my own needs first, after all, and what I want is to get out of the pickle I'm in. I want all of this tumor out of my body, I want to live a long, healthy life. I want a cure. I think about being rid of this tumor—if it were gone, would I miss it? Amazingly, I realize that there is a part of me that has identified this myeloma as me and doesn't want to let go. Hey, this is nutso, you don't want to accept this alien invader, you can give it up. I remember how I felt when I was pregnant, nauseated for months, rage at having my body taken over by an alien alternating with pride in creating a miracle. The pride and acceptance won out, but this is different. I can't let myself get comfortable with my myeloma, give it a home in my self. I want it out.

I think about a treatment Anne mentioned in passing, something she's going to find out more about. In England, some doctor has reported excellent results in giving very high-dose intravenous Alkeran to patients, enough to nearly totally obliterate their bone marrow, and then keeping them in isolation for weeks until the marrow "comes back." Ten percent died of overwhelming infection before the marrow recovered. The others are doing well, but it's only been about a year and a half.

I picture myself in the hospital that long. Could it be a private room? Would it have to be an intensive care unit? Could we do it in New York? If not, would I be willing to go to England? I think I'd go anywhere, but home would be better. Would it be a sterile bubble, no books, no visitors? When could we start? My mind whirls with the possibilities.

I must talk to Anne, tell her I want to do something

definitive right away. Why wait? Start in August; I don't have to go to my nephew's wedding, this is much more important. Start in August, I should be back at work by October, if I survive. I'm sure I'd survive. Ninety percent is pretty good odds, and I'm very strong. With antibiotics, I could withstand infection.

In Denver, we have to wait for the minibus to Vail. I have to talk to Anne. I find a pay phone some distance from where our group is waiting, dial her up, tell her secretary I'm calling from Colorado. Anne gets on. I tell her I've decided I want to go with something heavy as soon as possible, what has she found out? She has called some people but she hasn't hooked up with them; she's expecting them to call her back. She'll have more information in a week or so. I ask her if we could follow that British regimen at New York Hospital. Yes, we probably could, but let's wait a bit and see what there is. Anne, I really want to handle this soon, I don't want to prolong this anymore. I know how you feel, Cesca, but let's not leap into anything till we find out all the possibilities. Okay. Just relax, and have a good time in Vail, I'll talk to you when you get back.

In the minibus I realize that I want to tell Roger and Joan Mann about this now, before I undertake a radical treatment. I did a six-month fellowship in foot and ankle surgery with Roger three years ago. He is my mentor, and he and Joan have become close friends of ours. I want to tell them in person, not call them later and tell them on the phone. We arrive at the hotel and Roger and Joan wave to us from their terrace upstairs, tell us their room number. While we're checking in, there is a power failure due to a thunderstorm. The computer is down, sorry, we can't check you in, you'll have to wait in the lobby, it shouldn't be long. I leave Jim to check in, walk up the stairs to find Roger and Joan's room.

They have a suite, lit by the dark stormy light from the sliding glass doors that lead to the terrace. Their mood is light and gay. We sit down. Roger is opposite, way across the room, in darkness, the only light comes from the window-doors behind him; Joan is on the sofa a few feet away from me. What's happening, Roger asks cheerfully, how have you been? Not well, I respond. This is not going well, I start to cry, uncontrollably. I have a hard time getting the story out, but finally I do. They have never seen me like this, upset and out of control. Joan is caring and concerned but doesn't apprehend. Roger is grim, tight, glum; he has the whole picture in the diagnosis.

I tell them I've been keeping this a secret, it's important to me that nobody know about it. I might go for some heavy-duty treatment soon, but I haven't figured out if I could keep that a secret. Meanwhile I'm able to work, and that's what I want to do. Roger agrees wholeheartedly, says he would just work until he didn't feel well enough to and then just stop. I haven't really pictured that scenario, being too sick to work but too well to die, disabled. Not for me, I don't want to be disabled, chronically ill. I'd rather die.

Meanwhile, though, I want to stay active in the Foot Society, and I don't want my friends in this group to know I'm sick, because they would write me off as far as doing jobs in the workings of the organization, something I like to be involved with. Roger agrees. The lights come back on.

FRIDAY, JULY 18, 1986

The meeting is interesting, the morning passes swiftly. I don't give my talk till tomorrow, but I've rehearsed it enough not to worry too much about practicing some more. We decide to rent bicycles with the Manns and Bill Hamilton and ride them to Vail Village for lunch. On the bike path I turn my head back to see who's behind me and steer my front wheel off the edge of the track. I fall like a stone with my bike, jam my left elbow, and scrape the back of my right heel. It hurts like hell, but I am laughing; this must have looked just like the guy on *Laugh-In* in the yellow slicker, falling off a kiddie tricycle.

At lunch a little bit later, Jim notices the ugly scrapes on my heel. You are not supposed to get any cuts, he admonishes me. He's read the same booklet on chemotherapy, is worried that I'll get an infection. The Manns and Bill echo his concern. All right, all right, I'll handle it, I say, and leave for the ladies' room, irritated to be the focus of attention for something so trivial. I draw strange looks in the rest room with my foot in the sink, washing it off with soap and water.

After lunch we continue biking. I am very aware of the altitude, get short of breath easily. Bill's bike loses the chain and we can't go on. I am relieved. It was enough exercise for me, but I wasn't going to be the one to stop.

SATURDAY, JULY 19, 1986

My talk on problems of the second metatarsophalangeal joint goes very well, and I am pleased that I had been able to put it together while I had so much going on last month. A friend tells me he's editing a special edition of an orthopaedic monthly periodical and would like me to write my talk up for an article. I agree, thinking it won't be too difficult because it's really already done.

In the afternoon we suddenly join the rafting trip. It's been dry lately, so the water shouldn't be too high, quite safe. It is, but it isn't boring. In some places it's exciting, real white water. That's where they have a photographer ready to immortalize the event. The pictures are developed and blown up, suitable for framing, at dinner. Naturally, we buy the one that shows us clinging to the raft with glee, white water spraying all around us. This will be something for me to look at while I'm in the hospital, a reminder of a time when I could do exciting things.

I realize that I haven't kept my agreement with Anne that I won't do anything but rest and maybe shop in Vail. Well, I did shop a little. The only thing that I had in mind that I needed was something to wear in the hospital, and I found a couple of nightgowns, a hundred percent cotton, that are actually pretty too. Cotton is very absorbent, good for my night sweats. I'm still soaked at night. Pink. Yes, I can be pretty in pink with my wig in the hospital. Shit.

WEDNESDAY, JULY 23, 1986

After doing a couple of cases, I drive over to New York Hospital for my appointment with Anne. Get my bloods drawn, wait to see her. I hope she's got some good stuff for me, something better than the M2 protocol.

We sit at the round table in her office, drink the coffee I brought us. She's talked to a number of experts around the country. I grab some paper off the table, start to make notes while Anne rattles off the results of her many phone calls.

Anne begins. The thing that's had the longest track record is bone marrow transplant from a sibling donor, an allogeneic transplant. We don't even know if I have a match with one of my siblings, but even with an identical match, there are big problems. The risk of death is quite high: twenty-five percent die, either from infection because of immunosuppression necessary to allow the foreign bone marrow to engraft, or from graft-versus-host disease, where the transplanted cells, the graft, attack the recipient, the host, as a foreign presence, and therefore one to be destroyed. A double-edged sword. Lately efforts have been directed at reducing the culprit T-cells in the graft marrow so there is less graft-versus-host disease. Probably too extreme a solution for me at this time, Anne concludes. I go along with that.

She goes on. The group in Seattle that does the most sibling bone marrow transplants has done identical twin transplants. That has been quite successful. One twin has been well for about seven years with no relapse at all, except that she still has a "spike" in her protein electrophoresis, a sign that she is producing too much of one particular protein, a sign that the malignant focus is still there. That's very nice, I say, but I didn't happen to come with an identical twin, very inconsiderate of my parents.

Anne continues, looking over her scribbled notes. A noted myeloma expert in Tucson is currently working on various regimens of chemotherapy alone, but does not consider what he is doing to be strikingly innovative. He's getting about three-year median survival. He recommended some other centers and people.

Okay, who else? Anne glances at her list again. At the M. D. Anderson Cancer Center in Texas, a senior researcher in myeloma and a younger colleague have the most aggressive chemotherapy protocol. Mostly the younger guy is doing it. Called VAD, for vincristine (peripheral neuropathy), adriamycin (heart damage), and dexamethasone (high-dose steroids, lose my hips), it was initially developed for nonresponders, patients whose myeloma did not respond to more conventional and less dangerous chemotherapy. Now they're using it for initial treatment of previously untreated patients. They give four to six cycles of VAD, a four-day hospital admission each cycle, get the patient into remission, then give them their own marrow back after high-dose Alkeran and total body irradiation. So far they've done five patients, all have survived, the longest is eight months out so far. What about their spike? Anne doesn't know. But if they give them back their own marrow, isn't that like giving them back their disease? This one doesn't sound too hot. Lots of dangerously toxic drugs, a shotgun approach, blast everything to hell and gone, maybe me in the process.

I wouldn't be eligible for this protocol because I've already been started on the M2 program and have received two cycles of that. But the younger guy was very interested in my case, specifically in getting hold of my malignant plasma cells so he can grow them in culture and study their kinetics, how fast they grow, what slows them down. What? Travel down to Texas for a painful bone marrow just so this guy can study it? Forget it. Anne looks as uncomfortable as I feel with this outfit.

Then her face softens, she says she's spoken with the chief honcho at the Dana-Farber Cancer Institute. Where's that? In Boston. How come I haven't heard of it? They're a research-only hospital, not a big center like Memorial. They just take a few patients who are being treated on their research protocols. They started with childhood leukemia but have branched out into adult cancers, we've sent several patients up there for treatment and they've been very good with them, they really do a nice job. I can tell she likes them.

Anne continues, without notes now. He said they haven't done any autologous marrow transplants on myeloma patients yet, but they have a young researcher, Ken Anderson, who has just recently developed a monoclonal antibody against the plasma cell and may be gearing up to do a program to treat a marrow in remission with antibodies outside the body and then give it back after getting rid of the rest of the marrow in the body somehow. The key thing here is you get your own marrow back, so there's no problem with graft-versus-host disease, and the marrow you get back doesn't have tumor cells anymore. I perk up, this sounds really interesting, a very specific treatment, not a shotgun approach. Anne hasn't talked to Ken Anderson yet, but the chief honcho said he'd talk to him and Anne thought she'd probably hear from Ken soon, or she would call back.

Anne finds the third page of her scratch paper. There's another group that may be starting something similar. The myeloma maven at Johns Hopkins is gearing up to start a protocol of taking a remission bone marrow, treating it outside the body with strong chemotherapy, a derivative of Cytoxan, and then destroying the remaining marrow in the standard ways with chemotherapy and radiation and giving back the treated marrow. This sounds interesting, too, but what about the effect of the chemotherapy on the cells you want to transplant? How do you know if the chemo was enough to get rid of the malignant plasma cells in the marrow you give back? What if some of them are "resting" when they get drenched in poison, don't take it up, and survive to grow again in the transplanted marrow?

We both shrug; Anne moves on. There's another radical treatment that has a longer track record. A guy in England has been treating new cases of myeloma with very high-dose intravenous Alkeran, which nearly totally wipes out the marrow, and the patients stay in the hospital for four to six weeks and wait till the marrow regenerates spontaneously. Yes, I remember, Anne had mentioned this one to me before. Ten percent died. Better than the twenty-five percent mortality of sibling transplants. The only fly in the ointment here is that Dr. Kyle of the Mayo Clinic, the grandfather of myeloma lore, the guy who wrote the review article that stimulated me to seek something more aggressive, told her that one of their patients had recently had a relapse, so maybe it wasn't going to work out long-term.

That's about it, Anne finishes. I look at her. What did Dr. Kyle recommend? He likes a specific treatment, doesn't favor the aggressive VAD approach, thinks the M2 regimen is the one to stick with till it doesn't work anymore. The guy at Johns Hopkins isn't ready yet to get his study going, thinks M2 is fine in the meantime, it'll be several months at least before he's geared up for a clinical trial.

What do you like best, Anne? She's been trying very hard to present all these alternatives in an equal light. From your body language, Anne, I get that you're no more comfortable with the Texas outfit than I am. I think you like Dana-Farber's idea best, and I think I do too. It's so elegant, such a silver bullet. Just take out the bad cells and leave the rest. Or maybe a belt and suspenders would be better—combine both antibody and chemotherapy treatment of marrow outside the body. Anne looks doubtful. Yeah, I guess no one would want to mess up his research protocol with two experimental variables; if it works, no one would know which part of the treatment was responsible.

But what about my own immune system? If my marrow has no plasma cells, then I don't make antibodies anymore; would I be trading myeloma for something like AIDS, jumping from the frying pan into the fire? I don't know, Cesca, that's something you'll have to ask them.

You like how they've treated your patients, right? Yes,

they take very, very good care of them. They have a real system established, really manage the infections and transfusions well, can get the patient through the dangerous part, and the patients say everyone is nice to them up there. I can tell Anne is impressed.

What shall we do now? I'll be in touch with this guy at Dana-Farber and see if we can set it up for you to meet with them. Meanwhile, I think you should stay on the M2 regimen, and the next one is next week. We make arrangements for blood tests Tuesday, chemo Thursday, if the white count is okay.

When I drive home, I feel both elated and depressed. Elated that there may be something there for me, something that may halt the inexorable progression of this disease. Depressed at the realization that I may have to give up a lot. My freedom. I'd have to stop work for a month at least, maybe even six weeks. That's a long time. A long time cooped up in a small room, like a caged animal. I'd probably go nuts. It would be like going to jail. And how can I keep that kind of disappearance a secret? A long vacation, I guess, tell people I went to Italy to visit my family, hike in the Alps. I am focused on getting this miserable episode behind me as soon as possible, September maybe.

At home I tell Jim about the possibilities, referring to my notes, rehashing my whole conversation with Anne as we sit on our king-sized bed. He follows my recital intently, his dark, intelligent eyes unblinking as I discuss the risks, the possibility that some form of radical treatment might kill me. I tell him I want to give it my best shot, everything I have. He is grim, yet tells me he's there to support whatever I want to do. We hold hands, silent in our mutual understanding of what a long separation means. Not only will I be cooped up in a hospital, but I may be very far from home too. Maybe it won't be so bad, I say. Remember when I went to California for the fellowship with Roger for six months? I remember how we were all geared up for a horrendous time, and it turned out to be not bad at all, fun in fact, with all of us shuttling back and forth between the coasts on weekends and vacations, so we weren't apart for more than three weeks at a time. But that was then, and this is now, and the stakes are quite different.

I sense that he is not hopeful, but resigned. Resigned to losing me, resigned to my dying. He knows I will die, and has given up hope. I feel angry about this, but I can't bring it out, cannot offer hope when I feel guilty for being sick, for being so out of control of my life that this disease snuck up on me somehow when everything was going so well, when I finally had my life together.

WEEK OF JULY 26, 1986

Gradually I tell a little nexus of friends apart from work, maybe half a dozen, who share the secret and will be there for me to talk to, draw support from, and that feels a bit better. Actually, I don't want to talk about it much, although almost nothing else occupies my thoughts. It's with me all the time, except when I see patients, or operate, or watch the Mets play. Thank God for the baseball season, especially this season. The Mets are on a roll, and I identify strongly with their surge. If they can win, maybe I can win.

I notice that I'm so lost in my self-absorption I'm getting careless about simple things, like not getting run over by a bus. Missed me by inches, can't imagine what I was doing, standing there off the curb, vaguely waiting for the light to change. Did I want to get squished by a bus? Maybe that would be easier than facing all this mess, going through all this radical stuff, and what if it doesn't work? No, that's no way out, stepping in front of a bus. Be careful, don't do yourself in when you're not paying attention. I think about how we as orthopaedists have a sense that patients who have serious accidents are, as a group, more depressed, more preoccupied perhaps, than similar people who manage not to get injured. Are they trying to do themselves in, or do they have no attention span left for protecting themselves from ordinary dangers? I don't knew, but I resolve to be extra careful crossing streets. Tempting as it seems to end it all swiftly, I decide I don't want to do that, no, not really. Anyway, it might not work, and if it did, and it looked like suicide, there goes the life insurance. I don't want to go out that way, I want to fight to the end.

I think a lot about a guy we knew who threw himself a huge fortieth birthday party and then shut himself in his garage, reclined on a mattress by the exhaust pipe of his Mercedes, and died breathing the fumes. Speculation was rampant initially that he had some dread disease he couldn't face, but then it came out that he had been involved in a financial scandal and chose this way out. Yuppie hara-kiri. It made me angry. If he wanted to die so much, how come he didn't have myeloma?

I've noticed a strange thing: used to be that when I was falling asleep, just before I went under, I would get an overwhelming sense of myself all alone, totally isolated in a huge universe, a void, and I would have a feeling of dread, almost panic, at being so alone, so separate, in a place beyond the reach of all relationships. The funny thing is that it doesn't happen anymore, hasn't since I got sick. Now it's me and my myeloma, no void anymore.

On Tuesday I get my bloods checked again to see if we are go for chemo on Thursday. I'm pretty sure we will be.

*   *   *

The new housekeeper starts this week. We haven't had a housekeeper since Mrs. Taylor died over a year ago. But Jim and I decided we needed some help, we were struggling to keep up with the little things like shopping for food, laundry, picking up the dry cleaning and shirts, changing the sheets. I found a woman who was a friend of my sister's housekeeper, no Mrs. Taylor, but we'd give it a try. I showed her around the apartment, left elaborate lists. More trouble to write this out than do it yourself, I grouse to myself.

Coming home that evening, the place is neat and shiny, dinner is prepared, ready to be nuked in the microwave. Nice. A big relief, we've really needed a wife. Food doesn't taste too good, though. Maybe she can follow my recipes.

The blood tests were fine, white count up to a whopping 5, hemotocrit 38.8, nearly normal. What a difference! No wonder I'm doing better on the cross-country machine, up to about four kilometers now that I've got some hemoglobin to carry the oxygen around. And the back pain and sciatica are entirely gone, even off Feldene. Progress is being made.

Chemo session three goes smoothly on Thursday. I have plenty of time, having canceled my office hours for the morning. This cycle I can take less prednisone, just one week at 60 milligrams a day, then taper rapidly to nothing over three days. I am happy to be off prolonged steroids. After the full effect of this cycle, in about a month, we should get a bone marrow, Anne says, just to see where we stand after three months of treatment. I agree somewhat reluctantly, my hope that it's all gone dampened by my anticipation of another painful test. Speaking of tests, Anne, can we back off a bit on these weekly blood tests, maybe stretch it out to two weeks? Sure, you've been doing well, we don't have to look at it every week. Good, it's a real drag to drive over here and park so often.

What about the people up in Boston? Anne hasn't been able to talk to Ken Anderson yet, he's on vacation, should be back next week sometime. Hang in there. Okay.

WEEKEND OF AUGUST 1, 1986

A nice three-day weekend, especially nice because it's J's birthday and we can celebrate it with him for once. He's sixteen, old enough to drive, a real milestone. I spend some time with J in the big parking lot of one of the barns, giving him practice driving our old stick-shift '75 Volvo station wagon. Okay, clutch down, brake down, now ease off the brake and gently engage the clutch, then push the accelerator a bit. Okay, Mom, white knuckles on the steering wheel. Jerk, stall. Again, just easy now. Jerk, stall. Finally, a giant lurch forward. I grab the wheel, Hey, don't forget to steer! I can only take an hour of this, but he does get better, drives well enough to get us home into our own driveway. J concedes it's not as easy as it looks. It's just practice, J.

Every time we drive into Litchfield from our house, we pass the cemetery. I stare at the neat stone walls, the monuments within obscured by a thick line of tall fir trees. Mother told me recently that she bought a large plot a while back, "for the family." I wonder if she did this recently, for my benefit, or if she had already done it and is only now telling me about it, but I don't want to ask, don't want to confirm that she's given up on me too. She says it's very pretty, very peaceful. I know she'd show it to me if I say the word. I don't. No, don't want to look at it.

What about Burial Island? I ask her. I thought that was going to be the family place. Years ago my parents made an artificial lake in a spring-fed swamp below the fields and orchards planted with daffodils; it has a small island with a few artfully arranged granite boulders and scrubby evergreens. Daffodils bloom there in the spring. We've always called it Burial Island because we thought that would be a lovely place to scatter our ashes. We can't use it, it's against the law to scatter ashes anyplace you want, Mother says. Oh.

So I look at the outside wall of the cemetery as we go by, and cry, anticipating my funeral. I used to hold my breath when I went by a cemetery, all the kids did it on our day-camp bus, one big collective gulp, hands pressed against our mouths, then a big sigh as we got beyond it. Sometimes the bus driver teased us, slowing down so it was hard to hold on for the whole time it took to pass by. This cemetery was always the easiest one, not much road frontage.

But the Thompsons have a family plot too. Jim's mother's parents are there, and his aunt, and I think Jim's parents plan to be buried there, at least that's my assumption, we've never discussed it. I think Jim would want to be buried there, so maybe I should too. Would I want to be the only one in the Morosani plot? Would I be disloyal to my family to get buried in the Barlett and Thompson plot? Would Jim want to be buried next to me in my family's plot? Maybe that's a moot point, maybe he'd have another wife by then, I hope so, other ties. These permutations and divided loyalties are too much for me, I can't decide. I don't want to think about it, let them decide when I'm gone. The best way to avoid this dilemma is not to die.

MONDAY, AUGUST 4, 1986

I talk to Bill Hamilton about my progress, nothing short of fantastic. The recent IgG level was down to 3635, from close to 11,000. Never mind that high normal is around 1500, this is stupendous response to the chemo. Bill says that's really great, somewhat unenthusiastically, then volunteers some information reluctantly, saying he's not sure he should tell me this. Sure, I say, we can be honest with each other. Well, seeing as he didn't know beans about myeloma, he used his computer modem hookup with a medical literature search and called up some medical review articles and printed them out at home. Seems that people with a very rapid response to chemo don't have such a great prognosis, nobody knows why. Strange, I say, I never heard that before. I guess I'll have to ask Anne. God, I think, don't tell me I'm doing too well for it to last. Here I am working on getting rid of this, egging my white cells on to blast those blue babies whenever I think of it; am I overdoing it?

THURSDAY, AUGUST 7, 1986

Anne has some good news. She has talked to Ken Anderson about my case, and he is indeed gearing up to start autologous bone marrow transplantation for multiple myeloma, and she'll send him a copy of my records. He would like to meet with me. Great, what's his number, I'll call him up.

While I have Anne on the phone, I tell her about the review article Bill told me about. Does the fact that I'm doing so well mean my prognosis is worse? Anne seems perplexed, says she's never read or observed that, it's news to her. Besides, she adds, you are doing very well, but it hasn't disappeared with one cycle. Okay, I say, I was just wondering.

I call Ken Anderson from the office, leave a message, and he returns the call that afternoon. He sounds young, interested, friendly, and polite. After a few brief amenities, we agree the best thing is for me to come up to Boston to go over everything. How's next week? Fine, he says, any day. I choose Wednesday, a patient just canceled surgery for that morning and now the OR is fully booked, so it's a free day, except for a small ambulatory case, hardware removal, that can easily be rescheduled. He says to meet him in the adult clinic area about ten, if that's not too early. No problem, I'll take the shuttle and be there in plenty of time.

He says he'll have them send me some forms to register as an outpatient. Send them to my home address, I say, don't send anything to my office, my secretary doesn't know anything about this. He asks me to bring up all my records, or get Anne to send them, including the X rays and the pathology slides from my original bone marrow. I better bring them with me, they could get lost in the mail. Also bring all your insurance information, the business office will need that. Okay. See you Wednesday, then. Yes, I'm really looking forward to it.

Now we're rolling! I tell Ruth, my secretary, that I have to be out of town on some dumb family business on Wednesday, and we'll have to reschedule the hardware removal. Ruth doesn't bat an eye, says, Sure, I'll see if we can do it Tuesday, she wanted it done as soon as possible, I'll tell her we got an opening sooner. Ruth is always so eager to make things go easily for me. I'm lucky to have her.

I call Anne. I'm going up to Boston on Wednesday. Very good, Cesca. He sounds very nice, I said. Yes, and he thought you'd be a very good candidate for his protocol when I told him about you. Well, he wants to check everything out, and I'll need to take up my X rays and records and pathology slides. No problem, I'll pull all of that together for you and you can pick it up, say, Tuesday. Good. And while you're here, you can get some blood tests so we'll have the latest information for them. Sure, it's about the right time for a test anyway.

At home in the evening, I call Karen, my cousin in Boston, the one who spent the night with us the day I got the bad news. I'm coming up to Boston on Wednesday to see a guy who has a radical protocol for my myeloma. Where? The Dana-Farber Cancer Institute, do you know it? Cesca, that's where Cox works! Cox Terhorst is the guy she lives with. That's where he works? I thought it was the Jimmy Fund or some think tank. His lab is in the Jimmy Fund building, but he's in charge of the molecular immunology department at Dana-Farber. Golly, I never made the connection. You know, we've been wanting to talk to you about talking to these people up here, but we didn't want to interfere, and you had enough on your mind when you were starting your treatment. But listen, you ought to talk to Cox, he knows more about this than I do, let me get him.

Cox comes on with his thick Dutch accent, So, Chess, how did you find out about this? Did Karen tell you? No, my doctor, Anne Moore, talked to everyone in the country to find out what was happening, and this sounds like the best thing to check out. What do you know about it? Waal, they've been doing these "marrow cleanups" for a few years, but I don't think they've done any yet on your disease. No, I know that, it's a brand new protocol designed by a guy named Ken Anderson. Do you know him? Sort of, he worked in a lab down the hall from me, seems nice, but I do not know him as well as some of the others, one in particular is a very good friend of mine. Say, when are you coming up? Wednesday, this coming Wednesday, about ten o'clock. Look, why don't you come to my office first, it's right across the street, and we can talk; I'll find out all I can in the meantime. That's great, Cox, thanks very much.

Karen gets back on, asks, Do you want to spend the night? No, I don't think so, I have to be at trauma conference at seven-thirty Thursday morning. Well, I won't be on call that night, why don't you have dinner with us and then take the late shuttle down, that would be fun. Yeah, that does sound neat, you pick a place. Okay.

TUESDAY, AUGUST 12, 1986

I can hardly contain my excitement about going up to Boston tomorrow. I've been thinking about nothing else since last week. During a long hiatus between my morning and afternoon operative cases I go over to New York Hospital, get a whole battery of blood tests, and pick up my X rays and MRI scan, the pathology slides for microscopic examination of my bone marrow, and a small envelope addressed to Ken Anderson. I'm dying to open it, but it's sealed and I can't. Oh, well, I know what it says anyway, I've been keeping track.

My first two operative cases are "come-and-go" cases, so the patients go home immediately after surgery and do not have to be seen in the hospital the next day. The last case is an inpatient, a fascinating problem of disabling pain in a professional basketball player's foot, probably around a tendon on the outside of his right foot. He had total relief of pain when I injected a tiny amount of local anesthetic in the sore area, a good sign that the problem is localized to that spot. Several months of conservative treatment had not worked, and he was unable to sign a contract for the coming year, so he was willing, indeed eager, for me to explore the area to see if the problem could be solved, and soon. I knew how he felt. A quick fix: I wanted one too. So I open his foot, find a little pea-sized inflammatory nodule hanging off the edge of his tendon, catching on the surrounding tissue with sideways motion of the foot. No wonder he couldn't run and jump. After removing the offending tissue and sending it to the lab for pathologic examination, I close the incision, immobilize the foot and ankle in a dressing, and tell him I'm sure we found the problem. Luckily, the tendons are intact, and I think you'll be able to play by October. I am pleased, he is thrilled. I tell him that I want to see him in the office on Monday and that one of my partners will check him in the morning, and if he feels okay he can leave the hospital then, otherwise I'll see him Thursday morning in the hospital, and for sure he'll be ready to go. Stay on the crutches till Monday. Okay, Doc, thanks.

Even though we had discussed it last week when we scheduled the case and my patient knew I wouldn't be there, I feel bad about leaving town the day after I operate. I go over to the office and find Drew, tell him about the case, and ask him to check my patient in the morning and discharge him if he's doing as well as I expect he will. I explain to Drew about the possibilities of the protocol, he understands it's important and is interested in what I'm going to find up there. So am I.

WEDNESDAY, AUGUST 13, 1986

I get up a little earlier than usual, six o'clock. A gorgeous summer day, almost cool. Take a cab to LaGuardia, decide on the Pan Am shuttle on the half hour, take the 7:30. This is easy, just stick the American Express card in the machine and get a ticket. The other passengers are well-dressed business executive types, both men and women, and I must look like one of them with my beige linen blazer, paisley skirt, silk blouse, and leather briefcase. No one would guess I'm a cancer patient, carrying dried bloody smears of my myeloma-filled bone marrow in my nice leather briefcase.

I have my seat all to myself, no one can see what I'm reading. I pull out the material Dana-Farber sent me yesterday in a discreet envelope labeled D.F.C.I., even our mailman wouldn't know I was getting mail from a cancer hospital. I am impressed by their sensitivity. Map of where the hospital is, booklet of information about the hospital. Information forms for billing and insurance.

What name shall I use? I don't want word of my case filtering down to New York from Boston, and I suspect that having my name bandied about will be unavoidable if it turns out that I am considered seriously for the research protocol. I'll use Morosani, I won't have trouble remembering my own maiden name, even though I've used Thompson for more than half my life. Also, people have a hard time with Morosani, can't spell it or pronounce it, it'll be much harder to remember, and no way for anyone to connect it to me.

I glance over the booklets, glossy public relations efforts. One focuses on hospital services and a patient's bill of rights, quite boring, and a smaller one tucked into the back flap of the larger one explains how the Jimmy Fund evolved in the late forties to support research and early efforts at treating childhood leukemias with chemotherapy, with which they have great success by now, over fifty percent overall, over eighty percent in some types that had been only five percent curable a generation ago. Recently the researchers had added adult forms of cancer to their hit list. Myeloma wasn't one of them, yet, and this is dated 1986. At least it mentions bone marrow transplantation and monoclonal antibodies.

The cab deposits me at my destination by 8:45. I'm way early for my appointment. The building is a high-rise modern hospital. Across the street I see an older brick building with THE JIMMY FUND BUILDING carved in stone. That's where Cox works. There is construction scaffolding surrounding it, that's right, Cox said to use the side door because of the construction, and his office is on the third floor. I make my way there, and on the third floor find a blue-jeaned young man, probably a Ph.D. in typical research garb, who directs me to Cox's office.

Cox makes room for me on a broken-down old arm-chair, and I look around. The room is anarchy itself, books and papers in disheveled piles all over the place, the wall in front of his desk decorated with snapshots of Albert Einstein at various ages. Cox is dressed as casually as the other researchers wandering around, jeans and a wrinkled shirt. Lean and handsome, with gold-rimmed glasses, Cox reminds me of Jim. Looking at him, it's hard to believe he's one of the big shots here, sought after by other major cancer centers, but he is. Different uniforms for different jobs.

He's been checking out this marrow cleanup this past week, and it sounds interesting—totally out of his field, of course—but it also seems somewhat . . . radical. Yeah, I say, but I'm looking for an approach that could work. He advises me to ask a lot of questions, talk to several people up here, not just Ken. Okay. He pulls out a plastic folder and hands it to me. Here are some recent papers the transplant group has published on their results using monoclonal antibodies to clean up marrow in patients with lymphoma, and a copy of the new research protocol using this method against myeloma.

The research protocol! This is the document that details the experiment in recipe fashion and provides the justification for possibly fatal human experimentation to the watchdog committees that protect potential patients from unduly zealous or ill-advised interventions. How did Cox get this? I look it over, it has my undivided attention. Do you mind, Cox, if I read this right now? I'd like to read it before I have my meeting with Ken. Sure, sure, I have some stuff to do.

Over thirty pages long, it's hard reading, both emotionally and intellectually. I race through, knowing I'll read it again and again, but I want to get the whole picture as fast as I can. It's dated July 10, 1986. Gee, that's after I started to push Anne to find something new. This is really hot off the Xerox.

They call it "Intensive Combined Modality Therapy for Multiple Myeloma." Patient eligibility: age 18–60 years, okay; histologic diagnosis of multiple myeloma, plasma cell leukemia, and/or plasmacytoma, okay; plasma cell phenotype: PCA1 +. Now, what's that? I wonder. Cytoreduction—I guess that's reducing the number of tumor cells—with conventional chemotherapy to a complete response of less than 5 percent involvement with myeloma histologically, i.e., on microscopic inspection of the bone marrow—that would be pretty good; mine was 95 percent in May, I wonder what it's down to now?—and phenotypically—there's that word again, what the hell is that?—no nitrosurea or procarbazine—unfamiliar names, some form of chemo?

Protocol therapy is listed as, first, bone marrow harvest (how do they do that?) of autologous (that's my own, not a sibling's) marrow treated with monoclonal antibodies and complement (an immune factor that aids in the destruction of cells) in vitro, i.e., out of the body, to purge tumor cells; and, second, intensification (that's the oncologist's nice way of saying a humongous blast of chemo), a sequence of days of melphalan, which is my unpronounceable Alkeran, 70 milligrams per square meter intravenously. That's one huge dose for me; so far I've had 8 milligrams orally a day in my chemo regimen, and intravenous is stronger than oral dose usually, and I'm two square meters, so I would get 140 milligrams intravenously in one day, let's see, 8 into 140 is about 17, wow, this is close to twenty times what I've seen so far of Alkeran! And that's just the first day, the second day I get the same dose all over again. Then total body irradiation for three days in a row. And on the sixth day, reinfusion of autologous bone marrow, which has been treated with monoclonal antibodies and complement. And on the seventh day she rested. So all the treatment is in the first six days. So what takes so long?

I read on, skim the introduction, flip back and forth to the references cited to check where the information was coming from. "There will be an estimated 10,400 new cases of multiple myeloma in 1986," from the *Cancer Journal for Clinicians,* 1986. So there are a lot of other people in my boat. "Over the last two decades, there have been few advances in the understanding of myeloma or of its normal cellular counterpart, the plasma cell." That checks out, no one seems to know where it comes from. "More important, new therapeutic approaches have not led to cures, and all patients with multiple myeloma therefore succumb to their disease," from *Cancer Treatment Review,* 1981. Shit, there it is again in black and white. I know it, that's why I'm here, but reading it put like that makes me cry, again.

"This protocol describes a treatment program for patients with multiple myeloma, plasma cell leukemias, and plasmacytomas based upon the sensitivity of myeloma cells to high-dose alkylating agents and irradiation. The proposed escalation of drug dose"—I'll say!—"and total body irradiation can be employed only if: 1) this more aggressive therapy can be tolerated by the patient; and 2) tumor-free bone marrow is available to facilitate hematopoietic (blood-cell-forming) reconstitution after therapy." Yes, there has to be a way to survive the treatment. "Although myeloma usually occurs in older individuals . . . the younger patients (age thirty to sixty years) would be candidates for and tolerate higher doses of chemoradiotherapy." I'm on the younger side of the young group, and otherwise healthy.

"Tumor-free marrow to facilitate hematopoietic reconstitution could be provided from tissue-matched donors, but such donors are available for only forty percent of patients." We don't know yet if I have a match with one of my four brothers and sisters, we're going to check that out next week. "The use of autologous bone marrow requires methods to purge tumor cells, since myeloma is a disease intrinsic to bone marrow." Yes, of course, it makes no sense at all to give back marrow that still has tumor cells in it, like one of those regimens Anne described to me last month; we rejected that concept.

"In this protocol, we propose to use monoclonal antibodies directed at antigens expressed on the malignant pre-B, B, and plasma cells"—what are pre-B and B cells? what do they have to do with plasma cells?—"together with rabbit complement"—a protein harvested from rabbits that pops cells which have antibodies stuck on them—"to purge tumor cells while leaving behind normal hematopoietic stem (progenitor) cells. This treatment would permit autologous bone marrow rescue after high-dose chemoradiotherapy for multiple myeloma. This program would be modeled after the anti-B1 monoclonal-antibody-treated autologous bone marrow transplantation program for refractory B-cell lymphoma currently in use at the Dana-Farber Cancer Institute." Okay, so they've done this before with another disease. I wonder what the track record is, glance at the references; okay, Cox has a copy of one of these here for me, I'll read it later.

I keep reading the research protocol: "Clinical Course of Plasma Cell Dyscrasias (diseases)." "New therapeutic strategies are clearly necessary for the uniformly fatal plasma cell dyscrasias." There it is again—uniformly fatal. "In a study of 869 patients with myeloma, median survival was twenty months with only 66 percent and 10 percent of patients alive at one and five years respectively," from Kyle's 1975 Mayo Clinic report. Yeah, that's the one that really got me galvanized to do something, this guy's been reading the same stuff I looked at. "Complete remissions"—that's remissions, not cures—"have only rarely been reported." I skim on through details of failed chemo programs that produced initial reduction in tumor load, but rarely prolonged disease-free survival.

Some studies are cited that demonstrated that much higher than conventional doses of Alkeran or Cytoxan got pretty good but not permanent responses, suggesting that the more chemo you give, the better the result. Some other studies in patients with various cancers pushed the dose so high that bone marrow transplant had to be used to rescue the patient, because the worst thing high-dose Alkeran does is suppress the marrow. The other problems had to do with nausea, vomiting, diarrhea, and sores in the gastrointestinal tract. But it was shown that patients could survive the treatment.

A recent study combined high-dose Alkeran with total body irradiation for other cancers, and with bone marrow transplantation, the patients survived the treatment. High-dose Alkeran was used for myeloma with untreated autologous marrow, and the initial response was good, but the tumor came back right away from the transplanted cells, and no irradiation was used.

Now I'm getting confused. What does this mean? I guess no one has used high-dose Alkeran, and total body irradiation, *and* treated autologous marrow transplantation in myeloma before, but various combinations of high-dose Alkeran and irradiation have been used enough to show that patients can survive this attack, and if they are rescued with treated bone marrow, then maybe it will work. Clearly it doesn't work if the marrow isn't treated.

I skip over the next section, "Immunologic Studies of Myeloma." I can tell right away it's too complicated to figure out fast, it seems to be the story of how the antibodies they use were selected, very technical. I'll go back to this later. The bottom line seems to be that they have decided it will take three different antibodies, which they call anti-CALLA, anti-B1, and anti-PCA1, to knock out the malignant cells in the marrow.

The objectives of the protocol, what they are setting out to prove with this experiment, are listed:

> *1. To determine whether treatment of autologous bone marrow with anti-CALLA, anti-B1, and anti-PCA1 monoclonal antibodies can effectively*

purge antigen-bearing malignant cells without inhibiting or delaying engraftment.

So they want to find out if treating the marrow will prevent it from taking okay when they give it back. Okay, I hadn't thought that would happen, but it could be a big problem if the marrow didn't come back. I'd die.

> *2. To specifically delineate hematologic engraftment and immunologic reconstitution in patients who are treated with chemoradiotherapy and the reinfusion of purged autologous marrow.*

What does this mean? I get it, they want to show that the marrow actually works like normal marrow when it comes back, actually makes all the cells it's supposed to, white cells and red cells, and platelets, and also provides the immune cells necessary for survival. This sounds like the essential question I asked Anne: would I be trading myeloma for an immune deficiency like AIDS?

> *3. To determine if patients with multiple myeloma who achieve a clinical remission after conventional chemotherapy can achieve a prolonged, unmaintained [i.e., no more chemo] remission or cure—*

There it is, they actually said it! They are going for a cure!

> *—by the additional treatment of intensive combined modality therapy (melphalan and total body irradiation) followed by autologous bone marrow support.*

This is the heart of the whole thing, the bold step, they put it out there, they're willing to try for a cure. I want in.

They are going to be very choosy, I read in the next section, "Selection of Patients." Besides what was listed on the front sheet, there are further refinements. I try to figure out if I'll measure up. "No co-morbid disease, especially of the lungs, liver, and heart." They list some criteria and I check it out against what I know about my physical condition. My liver and kidney function are okay by their numbers. I'm pretty sure my heart and lungs will check out, given the kind of exercise I tolerate.

"Multiple myeloma documented by morphology and reactivity of tumor cells with anti-PCA1." What does this mean? Morphology means how the tumor cells look under the microscope. That's reasonable, to demand that the diagnosis is established before treating the disease so radically. That's why I brought my original diagnostic pathology slides with me. But what does reactivity with anti-PCA1 mean? The next page tells me the answer: another biopsy will be necessary in addition to the original diagnostic tissue. Well, we were going to do another biopsy this month anyway.

"No more than three isolated lytic bony lesions may be evident." I'm in good shape here, I have no bony lesions at all. Why three? I wonder. Isn't that kind of arbitrary? No matter, this requirement doesn't exclude me.

"Conditions for patient ineligibility." More reasons to exclude people from the study. Heart attack within six months, oversize and therefore unhealthy heart, cardiac arrhythmia, or irregular heartbeat. None of this applies to me; I'm glad my chemo hasn't included drugs that hurt the heart, that could knock me out of the study. Previous radiotherapy to pelvis or spine; I'm okay there. Concomitant malignancy—I guess that makes sense; you can't treat one tumor and get any sense of how the treatment works if another tumor may do you in. Pregnancy—that must be pretty rare in the age group that myeloma. An active infectious process—that makes sense; the treatment wipes out your immune system for a while, so there's no point starting out with a disease that could overwhelm you. Be off prednisone when the treatment starts—probably the same rationale, minimize immune suppression caused by prednisone.

"Prior treatment." They'll take anyone who has achieved a complete remission by conventional therapy. "Since myeloma is incurable with any current conventional chemotherapy"—it's getting easier to read this—"patients do not have to relapse after prior therapy to be eligible for this protocol." Good, I could start this as soon as I'm in remission. And it's okay to have had radiation to nonmarrow bone sites if it doesn't add up to too much for the normal tissue when the total body irradiation is added in. Again, this doesn't apply to me.

In the next section, "Treatment Plan," they suggest several forms of chemo to achieve complete remission. My M2 protocol is not one of them. Also, "nitrosureas or procarbazine may render the patient ineligible for entrance onto this protocol since they are known to be toxic to bone marrow stem cells." Okay, so they don't want to transplant cells that have been suppressed in growth potential by prior treatment, it might prevent the marrow from taking. Nitrosurea is ringing a bell for me—is BCNU a nitrosurea? I can't remember.

"Bone marrow will be harvested under general anesthesia from the iliac crests after the completion of conventional chemotherapy." How much do they take? Two cups? A gallon? How much is enough? How about getting some marrow from other bones?

I skip over the details of how they sort the cells and treat them with the antibodies but note that they try to keep it sterile, check it for bacteria and fungus contamination, and have a way of checking that they haven't killed the cells. Then they freeze the harvested marrow, thaw it when it's time to give it back.

This is interesting: "For the first five patients entered on this protocol an aliquot"—what's an aliquot?—"of marrow will not be treated with monoclonal antibody and will be cryopreserved (frozen) to serve as a backup should engraftment with the treated bone marrow be inhibited (white blood cell count less than 100 at day 19 after the transplant)." Sounds like an aliquot is enough marrow to do another transplant, so that would mean they'd have to get two transplants' worth of marrow when they harvest. So there's a fail-safe plan for rescue if the marrow doesn't take, but it wouldn't work for long; that other study has already shown that myeloma comes back very fast when untreated marrow is transplanted. I don't know if I'd want to agree to that. This is a way to make sure a patient survives the immediate transplant and doesn't die in the hospital. Maybe I'd rather take my chances and have the second batch treated and used to beef up the first batch. Go for broke.

"Intensification with melphalan and total body irradiation." More details of how they give the chemo and irradiation. I skip ahead. "Within twenty-four hours after completion of total body irradiation, patients will receive back their autologous bone marrow as a rapid intravenous infusion through a large-bore needle equipped with a blood filter." So that's how they do it! Just like a blood transfusion. I had pictured perhaps injecting the transplant with big needles into my pelvis, sort of a reverse bone marrow aspiration. This sounds much nicer, and not as painful. At least this sounds easy for me.

"Supportive therapy." Yes, this could be the hard part, I'm going to need support. "Anti-emetics as per routine." Drugs to make me not throw up. I think about how Compazine zonked me out. Specially treated red blood cell transfusions to keep my hematocrit higher than 30. I don't like the idea of getting other people's blood—a good way to get hepatitis, other viruses, AIDS. Specially treated single-donor platelet transfusions to keep my platelet count higher than 20,000. That's pretty low, lower than that and you could bleed to death, or have a fatal brain hemorrhage. But again, I don't like the riskiness of platelet transfusions, you can pick up the same diseases. This is strange:

NOTE: ALL BLOOD PRODUCTS ADMINISTERED AFTER BONE MARROW GRAFTING SHOULD BE IRRADIATED WITH 2000 RADS IN ORDER TO AVOID GRAFT-VERSUS-HOST REACTIONS.

So even other people's blood could attack me when my own immune system is suppressed. The last item on the supportive therapy is a prophylactic antibiotic, Bactrim, to be taken twice daily. To be taken to prevent what? Urinary tract infection? That's what Bactrim is usually used for.

"Toxicity." Yes, the part that makes you sick. This is the bad part that can happen in this protocol. "Profound and prolonged marrow suppression, which may prove lethal if the transplanted marrow does not engraft, with the nadir occurring seven to ten days after treatment and lasting seven to twenty-one days." Okay, there it is, this treatment can kill you.

"Severe GI toxicity with nausea, vomiting, mucositis, and diarrhea are possible." Not guaranteed, but possible. "Sterility is to be expected." This is not a problem for me, but does it mean menopause? "Interstitial pneumonitis may occur and may prove lethal." Uh-oh. Another way to go, I wonder why? "Cataract development is possible with total body irradiation." Golly, I need my vision pretty sharp to operate. Oh, well, cataracts can be fixed surgically.

A new section, "Required Data." Just before the transplant, a lot of tests have to be done to document that all the eligibility requirements have been met. Okay. During the time in the hospital, more daily and weekly blood tests are to be done. Many needle sticks, I guess. And many bone marrow tests for the first eighteen months after the transplant. Sounds like a lot of trips to Boston.

"Patient Consent and Peer Review." They agree to obey all the rules of the hospital, the National Cancer Institute, the State of Massachusetts, and the federal government that have to do with informed consent and having other physician peers review this protocol to make sure no unjustifiable experimentation occurs. A special informed consent must be signed by the patient.

"Statistical Considerations." I was never very good at statistics, so I don't think I'll get much out of this. "The principal objectives of this study are the evaluation of the toxicity and the efficacy of intensive combined modality therapy and autologous bone marrow support." So they want to see how sick it makes me, and if it works. "Toxicity will be monitored in terms of delay in hematologic reconstitution or other unexpected toxicities." I don't like this "unexpected" part, it feels like they've anticipated quite a lot. "Efficacy will be evaluable on the basis of disease-free survival and long-term survival." They plan to take fifteen patients into the study before deciding whether it works or not, unless more than two "evaluable" patients fail to engraft by six weeks after the transplant; if that happens, they stop the study and go back to the drawing board. This "evaluable" business is passing strange; a patient is not "evaluable" unless he survives to one month after the transplant. Does this mean a death before then doesn't count?

"A disease-free survival of at least six months will be considered to be clinically meaningful." To me, that's a drop in the bucket. If none of the first fifteen patients achieves this, the study will be stopped, but if even one patient makes it six months disease-free, they'll expand the study to a total of forty patients. The reasons for this are backed up with a bunch of statistical mumbo jumbo that is meaningless to me.

Appended at the back is the Dana-Farber Cancer Institute's informed consent: TRANSPLANT PREPARATIVE REGIMEN: MELPHALAN AND WHOLE BODY IRRADIATION. This is what I'd have to sign before I could enter the study. It seems to be the researcher's plain English version of all I've read so far. Most of it, I note as I flip through it, is a rehash of what I've just plowed through. I wonder if there's anything that hasn't been explicated so far.

Your disease, multiple myeloma, is currently in remission but has a high probability of recurring within the next few months to one year. Retreatment with chemotherapy at the time of relapse can be effective in obtaining yet another remission, but the ease with which this is accomplished and durability of second remission are both markedly diminished. The complete eradication of tumor leading to a cure is not thought to be possible for patients with multiple myeloma using standard chemotherapy.

Entering this study will make you a part of an experimental treatment program attempting to decrease the chances of your disease relapsing. In this study, you will receive short-duration, high-dose melphalan chemotherapy and radiotherapy. The radiation treatments will be given over the entire body at short intervals during a three-day period. Both chemotherapy and radiotherapy will be given in an attempt to kill every last tumor cell in your body. One of the side effects of this combined therapy is the destruction of your bone marrow cells, which are the blood-forming elements of your body found inside many of your bones. This lethal complication of combined treatments is avoided by removing some of your bone marrow ("the harvest") before treatment begins. Later your "harvested" bone marrow will be given back to you in a simple transfusion ("transplanted"). Your bone marrow cells will seek out their original bones and begin making blood cells.

Multiple myeloma, by nature, has the like-

*lihood of lodging cancer cells in your bone mar-
row. Therefore, your "harvested" bone marrow
will be treated to remove these tumor cells before
it is given back to you. Three monoclonal antibodies, anti-CALLA, anti-B1, and anti-PCA1 will
be used in treating your "harvested" bone marrow
following its removal from your body. Treatment
with these antibodies will then be done to kill any
cancer cells remaining in your bone marrow.
Your bone marrow will then be "transplanted"
back into you with an intravenous infusion and
will replace those normal bone marrow cells
which have been destroyed by chemotherapy and
radiation treatment.*

Okay for the big picture; the next few pages detail the
therapy from the patient's point of view and reiterate the
rationale for the treatment, namely, nothing else has
worked for long.

But the requisite reminder of alternatives is present,
what's in store for me if I don't elect this treatment:

*1. No further treatment at this time, but there is a
likelihood your disease will return.*

*2. Treatment with routine chemotherapy when
your myeloma relapses.*

*3. Surgery or radiation therapy might be utilized
to help control localized disease if and when your
tumor returns.*

*4. This protocol would be available to you after a
relapse only if you can get into remission a second time. It is likely that your disease will be
more resistant at that time to the kind of approach and treatment offered here.*

5. At any time, you may choose to receive only supportive care to relieve any pain or discomfort you may be experiencing.

At what point, I wonder, would it get so bad that I'd say, Stop the treatment, just give me morphine and let me die?

6. You are free to withdraw from the study without any prejudice at any time. To withdraw after initiation of therapy would be fatal.

Yes, once you get on the roller coaster, there's no getting off till the ride ends. I hate roller coasters.

There's a final grim reminder of possible problems: "The Dana-Farber Cancer Institute has no program for compensating patients or providing treatment for unanticipated medical injury arising from this research."

That's it, the whole protocol. My mind is reeling. I find it hard to connect all of this to me, yet there are little flashes that it could be me, in a totally new environment. This feels a little like reading school catalogues before September, picturing what it's going to be like. It was never what I had imagined, I wonder if this will be the same.

I better go over and register at the clinic, the appointment letter they sent said I was scheduled for noon, but to come about an hour and a half earlier and check in at the reception desk in the main lobby. Cox gives me his extension number, explains how to make an inside call so I can reach him when I'm done and we can get together for dinner.

Volunteers staff the reception desk, warm and welcoming. Please sit here in the lobby, someone will be with you soon. Sure enough, a woman in civilian garb calls out my name, escorts me into a room with a computer console. She explains she is a nurse who conducts registration interviews, they have a bunch of information they need to log in. We go through it, insurance, demographic information. I explain that I am using Francesca Morosani here, and my Connecticut address. Oh, are you recently married? No, hardly, it'll be twenty-two years this month, I'm just concerned about confidentiality. No one knows about my diagnosis and I want to keep it that way. She emphasizes that my medical records are private here. I'm sure they are, but the medical world is a very small one, and I'll feel better this way. When we finish, she points the way to the adult clinic.

I have quite a bit of time. I wander around the lobby, look at the huge oil portraits of the founders. Who was Dana Farber? I wonder. I soon find out there was no Dana Farber. This hospital has been named after Sidney Farber, a doctor who started chemotherapy for children over thirty years ago, and Charles Dana, a wealthy philanthropist who supported this effort financially. Dana hyphen Farber.

I find the adult clinic in the back of the main floor. White Formica counters, a small patients' sitting area with magazines, examining rooms all around. Everyone is cheerful and friendly, greeting patients and family members like old friends. The atmosphere is distinctly different from New York clinics, no one is harrassed, indifferent, or acting like they're being forced to do something that's not in their job description. A pink-coated volunteer is pushing a cart around, offering free coffee, tea, hot chocolate. Thank you, I'd love some coffee, black, please. I watch the doctors come and go. Some of the patients look sick, pale and yellowish, women with obvious wigs, young men with baseball caps over bald heads. I can't identify with them. At least I have my hair. I try to read my *New York Times*.

Dr. Thompson? I look up. I'm Ken Anderson. I stand up, tower over him. We shake hands, smiling. I am immediately struck by his resemblance to one of my best friends, same height, about five six, sturdy build, receding brown hair, clear light brown hazel eyes, twinkling, merry eyes, he's a pixie in a white coat. I like him instantly. He escorts me into a nearby room, and we each take a chair.

I reach into my briefcase. I have a lot of stuff for you. Good, he says. I hand him the slides, the large X-ray packet, and Anne's letter. He puts it all on another chair, takes up Anne's letter. Okay if I read this now? Of course. He reads swiftly, I watch him intently.

Okay, very good. He looks up. Can we go over your history together? Sure. We talk, I tell him the whole story, leave nothing out, shortness of breath skiing, the chest pain, the resolved back pain, the abnormal protein in August of '85 that nobody noticed at the time. We agree that the disease was there a year ago, progressed very rapidly for a myeloma. My rapid improvement since the plasmapheresis and the M2 chemotherapy regimen, my desire to knock this tumor out once and for all, my concern about the risks of years of low-dose chemotherapy, my willingness to give up my practice for a hospitalization of a few weeks, even a couple of months, to achieve this—I lay it all out.

Well, here's the scoop, Ken says, and starts to describe the autologous bone marrow protocol. I interrupt, reaching into my briefcase for the protocol, Actually, I've had the opportunity to read this quickly this morning, and I have some questions. He seems a bit surprised, but not unhappy, that I'm so prepared.

Over here, where it says no procarbazine or nitrosureas, what is that stuff, is it BCNU? Yes, now, here's the scoop, BCNU suppresses the stem cells, and we don't like to use it for patients who are candidates for marrow transplant because it might make their stem cells slow to come back, or unable to come back at all. Well, I've had three doses of BCNU so far, is that going to be a problem? He looks at my chemotherapy flow sheet, which Anne sent, frowns. It'll probably be okay, but we can talk to Anne about it. He's treading carefully here, I can tell he feels awkward about interfering in another doctor's management of my treatment. Maybe we can work out an adjustment, he offers, a modification of the M2 protocol. You mean drop the BCNU out of it? Yes, maybe increase some of the other agents. Well, we've already modified the standard protocol by giving me half the usual dose of vincristine because I need my peripheral nerves to operate, I wouldn't want to increase that one.

I noticed that the M2 protocol is not listed as a way to achieve clinical remission to qualify for the protocol, let's see . . . I point to the paragraph. You talk here about two different regimens: the high-dose vincristine, adriamycin, and dexamethasone one, and the high-dose Cytoxan one, and you say "patients will be treated with this therapy to achieve complete remission status prior to eligibility for this protocol." Is this a must? Do I have to switch to this to be eligible for the protocol? Anne has told me that this high-dose stuff could make me sick, unable to work, that I may even require hospitalization if I get a fever for a week or two of IV antibiotics, I wouldn't like that at all. Also, I go on, the one with the high-dose vincristine— The VAD protocol, Ken interjects. Yes, the VAD one, I have a lot of concern about all three drugs—the vincristine could knock out the sensation in my hands, the adriamycin could damage my heart, and the dexamethasone could knock off my hips, give me aseptic necrosis. All of these would really affect the quality of my life.

Ken shrugs sympathetically. Well, here's the scoop— I'm beginning to imagine that his nickname around here must be "Scoop" Anderson—getting into a complete clinical remission is the important thing, and if you are getting there on some form of the M2 regimen, even though we don't recommend that one particularly, the main objective is to get to complete remission status before we can go ahead with the autologous bone marrow transplant. When you get to that point, we would insist that you have a "consolidation course" of high-dose chemotherapy just before we plan to do the transplant and then let your marrow recover from that before we harvest it. Why is that? What's better than a complete clinical remission? Well, you can be in complete clinical remission, as we define it, with a normal protein level, normal hematocrit, and a normal number of plasma cells in your bone marrow, but we know the tumor is still there in some finite number of cells because the protein electrophoresis will still show an abnormal band, which indicates that there is too much of one particular protein being made by the malignant clone of cells. We can also use special antibody immunofluourescent stains on your bone marrow and identify the cells in a cell counter by how they flash, and see that they are monoclonal and therefore from the malignant clone. So the idea is that we want to reduce the actual numbers of tumor cells from the marrow as much as possible before we harvest it so we have a better chance of totally cleaning up the marrow when we treat it with the three antibodies.

I see, I say. Kick it when it's down.

I change the subject. Lemme ask you about the bone marrow harvest: how much do you take? Do you get it only from the pelvis? Have you ever thought about getting it from other bones too? No, we haven't done that, we just aspirate it from the iliac crests with multiple sticks. How much do you take? Oh, about a liter, as much as we can. I start to calculate, about 10 cc per aspiration, that's a lot of sticks. Yes, Ken says, probably hundreds. That's why we use general anesthesia. But we don't make that many holes in the skin. Once the needle is in, we can redirect it and get ten or twenty aspirations per skin stick. The pelvis must look like Swiss cheese when you're done. Yes, he concedes, it has a lot of holes, but they seem to heal up pretty fast.

It sounds like a pretty boring operation, just standing there aspirating for a couple of hours. True, Ken says, but two of us do it together, working on each side to make it go faster. That's a lot of continuous work for your hand muscles, don't they hurt? Yes, a little, but we get used to it.

You know, it seems to me that once you get a good marrow to harvest, you'd want to take as much as you could. Why not go for the marrow in the proximal and distal femur, the proximal tibia, the proximal humerus? Ken looks uncomfortable. I see the inside of all these bones when I do fracture work, it looks to me like there's a fair amount of marrow there too. You could get a whole bunch more good marrow if you go after it. That may be, Ken says. Look, I say, I know internists don't know very much about anatomy and don't want to go sticking needles through skin when they don't know if they'd be poking a nerve or an artery, but there are plenty of good orthopaedic surgeons up here who could scrub, too, and they'd know which approaches would be safe. Also, you could ream the long bones with the kind of instruments we use for fracture work, make a small incision, and then ream the intramedullary cavity. Well, we can talk about it, he says, it might be possible.

There's one other thing I want to tell you about the harvest operation that's not in the protocol. Oh, what? Well, venous access is very important during the time you're in the hospital. Yes, I think, I've already figured out there will be many needle sticks a day, and after a while all the veins wear out and it gets harder and harder to find one that can still be used for an intravenous line or blood drawing. What we use is Hickman catheters, and we get a surgeon to put two of them in while you're asleep, before we turn you over to harvest the marrow from the posterior iliac crests.

Yes, I remember back in 1981, they had started using these surgically implanted long-term Silastic catheters at Memorial Hospital. In fact, another resident in my group and I had brought this new idea to Special Surgery that year and convinced our attendings to let us put them in patients who needed six weeks of antibiotics for treatment of infected joints. I have to say we were as much motivated by our desire not to have to restart intravenous lines in the middle of the night when we were taking care of the patients as by the fact that life was much better for patients who wouldn't have trouble with daily painful IV starts in worn-out, inflamed veins.

But I remember also that it required a fair-size incision on the upper outer chest, dissection through the muscle to find the vein that led into the large subclavian vein, the one that lies right under the collarbone and empties right into the heart. You put the special Silastic tubing into the vein and thread it forward so it goes just above the heart. We used to check the position on X ray, to make sure it went to the right spot, didn't take a wrong turn and wind up in the neck. Then you tunnel under the skin in the fatty tissue over the muscle and bring the Silastic tubing out through the skin a few inches away in the center of the chest. There was a Velcro-like cuff at the exit point, just under the skin, that caused the tissue to scar around the tubing so it wouldn't move in and out, and that kept it from becoming contaminated or infected. With proper skin care, you wound up with an intravenous line that could last for months and could be used for blood drawing as well.

But you also wound up with permanent scars on your chest. Four big scars on my chest that would show in a bathing suit or evening dress. The exit scars would show in a V-neck blouse. I don't like it. I scar terribly, always have. I picture the dresses I won't be able to wear, the red one, the purple one, both with spaghetti straps. Oh, well, they don't fit me now anyway. This is the least of my problems.

How come two? Isn't one enough? Well, it's useful to have two because you may need antibiotics running in one and red blood cells or platelets in the other. It's more convenient. Also, sometimes one of them gets clogged and you can't draw blood back from it, so it's nice to have a spare. And sometimes when a patient has persistent fever, we culture the blood from the lines, and if we suspect that the line is infected we have to remove it, so again it's good to have a spare. Okay, I think, in for a dime, in for a dollar, forget the scars.

Ken goes on, You know, one of the things we have to check out is whether your marrow has cells that react with the antibodies we have. I figured this was in the offing. Yes, Anne and I were planning to do another bone marrow at the end of this cycle of chemo to see where we stand. It's a good idea to do it before the marrow is in remission. I brighten up. You mean you think it could be all gone! No, that's probably not the case, but I did see a guy not too long ago who's interested in this protocol, and his marrow has been treated so hard there's nothing left right now to react to the antibodies, so he's not eligible. So what's he going to do? Wait and see if the tumor comes back, and if and when it does, test it again against the antibodies.

Do you have time to do a bone marrow now? Yes, I reserved the room, I think we can go ahead. Ken turns me over to the nurse, who gets my weight and blood pressure and takes me to the bone marrow room, where I change into a hospital gown. They call them "johnnies" here, why I don't know. A technician comes in and sets up the slides. Ken comes in, says we should get both sides. Okay. It's not so bad, less painful than the last one, but still not so pleasant. Elastic tape is applied to the dressings. Okay, that's it, Ken says. You mean I don't have to lie here for half an hour? Ken is surprised. No, why? That's what they do at New York Hospital, something about preventing bleeding. Ken smiles. Well, I guess each institution has its own methods. And no signed consent here either, I add. Not yet, he says, but it may be coming.

Ken excuses himself to deliver the slides to the regular lab, and the specially treated aspirate of cells to his own lab for the special immunologic testing. He suggests I get some blood tests also. I had all those tests yesterday at

New York Hospital, how about if I call and get the results, that would be cheaper than repeating everything. Sure, that would be fine. We agree to meet back in the clinic area after he sees another patient who's been waiting to see him.

I find the pay phone in the lobby and dial up the lab on my credit card. Write down about twenty plus numbers. Everything looks good to me. Total protein is down to 7.4, that's the best yet, a big, big change from the 18 it was before. Albumin is part of that, normal at 4, and the other fraction of serum protein is the globulin part, and it's down to 3.4, normal. How about that! But these are gross tests, not the refined qualitative and quantitative serum protein electrophoresis test that takes a couple of weeks to get back from the lab. That's the test that really analyzes what the picture is with my immunoglobulins, the normal ones and the one that's off the chart, overproduced in huge quantities by the rogue malignant clone of plasma cells. It's funny to me. These cells are cancerous, exist in overwhelmingly huge numbers, yet each cell is just doing its job, what it's programmed by its DNA to do: make one specific immunoglobulin, or antibody, releasing small amounts of that one special antibody into my system, okay in and of itself, intended to be useful in defending against infection, but in the aggregate of trillions of cells, gumming up the works. I think of my close call with a potential stroke a couple of months ago. Phew, got out of that.

I return to the clinic area, sit down to wait for Ken. I think some more about my protein level being normal now. It wasn't a year ago. I pull out my little red diary, flip to the back where I write all my lab results. Yes, those tests I had a year ago after the dirty cut in the operating room. We paid no attention to that slight abnormality, we were looking for my liver functions, evidence of possible exposure to hepatitis from becoming blood sister to a drug addict with an infected hip, possibly with ARC, AIDS-related complex. The total protein had been 8, the highest limit of normal, but the globulin was 4.5, and the high normal was 3.5. I never focused on it then. Would it have made any difference? Surely I had myeloma then, I'll bet my marrow would have shown increased numbers of plasma cells then, probably about the same as it is now, whatever that turns out to be, if the level of excess protein is any indicator. Well, this protocol wasn't anywhere near ready then, so I can't say I've lost out on anything by a delayed diagnosis. Just months more misery. I'm glad I didn't find out then.

Ken returns, says, Let's go show your films to our radiologists. I trot after him, we wind our way down the stairs to a subbasement level, into a darkened room where X rays are being read out by a couple of guys, evidently a radiologist and a resident. We wait diffidently while they finish what they're doing. The tall one turns to us, Ken makes the introductions, subtly letting him know that these are my films we'll be looking at, but I'm one of them, another doctor, it's okay. We put all the films up on the mammoth light board, he studies them carefully, concurs with the previous finding of totally normal skeletal survey.

We put all the films back in the manila envelope, Ken hands him the other one. This is something new, a total body MRI. The tall one perks up, Gee, I've never seen one of those, I'll be happy to look at it out of interest but I don't think I can give you a reading, we don't have that technology here yet. We put the MRI films up, they look at it speechless. I fill in the void, pointing out the black lines of cortical bone, the mottled appearance of the marrow areas, thought to represent marrow infiltration with tumor, yes, ninety-five percent tumor involvement at that point. They are fascinated, shake their heads in amazement at the anatomical detail of the MRI scan. I sense they're ambivalent about this technology; on the one hand, you can see so much, on the other hand, a lot of what they know about reading conventional films could become obsolete.

It's hard to keep up in medicine. We gather up the MRI, thank them, and leave.

We return to the clinic area and find an unoccupied room where we can talk some more. Ken says the slides should be ready to read soon, the regular slides, not the special immunologic tests, that takes a day or so.

I look at Ken and consider him carefully; golly, he's so nice, so accessible, is he trying to snow me? I want a cure desperately—can I trust him? What does he want? He's created something that could make medical history if it works, that would be a peak experience for any scientist. Can he retain his clinical judgment? Would he risk my life foolishly? Can I trust him with my life? I better get to the hard questions.

I want to know, I say, how many deaths you've had. Deaths? Yes, Cox told me you've used essentially this same bone marrow cleanup on a couple of other diseases, so tell me how many people have died doing this tranplant? Two. Out of how many? About fifty in the relapsed B-cell lymphoma group. What did they die of? Ken looks distressed, as if remembering an unhappy time. One died of bleeding. We just couldn't keep his platelet count up, he became refractory to all platelet transfusions, just chewed up the platelets and they didn't work, Ken says, shaking his head sadly, even with all our special donors.

You know we have the biggest blood component bank in all New England, people come from all over to give blood here if we call them, Ken digresses now, happy to tell me something more cheerful. In fact, tonight we're having one of our annual parties for our volunteers. We're having a supper party on a boat in the harbor. I have to be there, one of the hats I wear here is as director of the blood component lab, and we're going to recognize our big givers. It makes them all feel like part of our family, and we'll have some patients who will talk to them about how grateful they are. It makes them seem real to the donors.

How do you get your donors? Mostly they are friends and family of past and present patients, they start giving when a loved one is in the hospital. We keep track of them, and when we need a special match for a certain patient, we call them. You'd be amazed how loyal they are, some people will drop everything and drive five hours down from Maine, say, to give platelets or whatever to a patient who matches them, someone they don't know. That is amazing, I say, what a gift to a stranger! That's why we try so hard to let them know they are appreciated.

Speaking of transfusions, I say, I'm not too keen on transfusions for obvious reasons. We feel the same way, we have very stringent tests for all our blood component transfusions. We match them very carefully, check for hepatitis and other viruses like CMV and, of course, AIDS. How's your track record with AIDS? Ken frowns. Not too bad, but when the AIDS test came out, we did go back and check and found one out of thousands of donor samples was positive for AIDS. We felt terrible about it, of course, but there was no test at that time, no one knew about the AIDS epidemic. I think our rate was less than a lot of the big regional blood banks, maybe because we have such a select donor group.

Well, my family is very eager to give blood for me, how about using their blood? They'd come up here for me, I'm sure. Ken is trying to be tactful. That's nice, he says, but we won't know them as well as some donors we've used for years, and sometimes family members are so anxious to give they forget to tell us things we need to know. I laugh. You mean, like they're homosexual, or Haitian, or IV drug abusers? He smiles. Well, yes. At any rate, he goes on, if we ever got into trouble matching your platelets, we'd have your siblings in reserve. Anyway, we do single-donor platelet transfusions routinely, so each transfusion of platelets is from only one donor, and there's less chance of developing a reaction against it, compared to the usual way of making a platelet transfusion from the pooled platelets of lots of donors. How do you get them? It takes a couple of hours of plateletpheresis from each donor. I remember my two sessions of plasmapheresis, am impressed at volunteers doing this to give away their platelets.

I realize we've gotten sidetracked. What about the other one? What other one? The other patient who died? Oh, he died of acute liver disease, an unpredictable complication. What happened? Well, we don't know what caused it, whether it was the chemotherapy he had—not the same that you'd have—or the total body irradiation. It's the only time we've had this complication, and it's been reported as a rare occurrence out of some other centers. What was it exactly, hepatitis? No, not serum hepatitis, something called VOD, venocclusive disease; the small central veins in the liver shut down, cause an acute liver necrosis. He shakes his head, helpless and sad-looking. I shudder inwardly—it's like being a duck in a shooting gallery, anything could strike me down. I shake it off, nonsense, no reason to think that will happen to me, look at all the others who haven't had that complication.

I change the subject. How long do you think I'd be in the hospital? Probably about a month, and then we'd want you to stay up here a week or so just in case you need more transfusions. Can't I get transfusions in New York? Well, to be frank, we like our patients to get our own blood, for all the reasons we've just discussed, plus all the special treatment the blood that we give post-transplant patients gets, special freezing and then irradiation to make sure you won't have any reactions to any stray donor white cells that could be mixed in with the red blood cells or platelets. Okay, that's reasonable.

Do I have to stay in one room all the time? Oh, yes, but a very nice room, you'll see. I'll show you the floor later, where the transplant unit is, the patients are in what we call reverse isolation. I think back to when I worked in the burn unit at New York Hospital, the serious burns— "crispy critters" we called them, to distance ourselves from the horror and pain of their injuries—were so susceptible to infection that we donned new gowns, gloves, masks, and hair covering every time we entered their rooms for any reason.

What kind of reverse isolation? Can I have visitors? Sure, you can have a few visitors, but everyone who goes in has to scrub up, put on a special gown, mask, and sterile gloves. Yes, it sounds like the burn unit, the memory is distinctly unpleasant.

Will I be sick? After the first couple of weeks, when everyone gets sick with the chemo and the radiation, but we have a pretty good program of medicine for that, I think the biggest problem for you is going to be boredom, cabin fever. Yes, I say, it sounds like jail. Can I have books? Sure. My computer? Sure, and there's a TV, and we have a VCR and a whole library of film tapes for you to choose from. Can I bring a radio, tapes? Sure, the nurses just wash the stuff you want to bring in with some special stuff, then it's okay. I picture myself getting caught up with a bunch of professional reading, maybe writing a clinical paper. No telling what I could accomplish with all that time available.

What about exercise? I could go nuts with no chance to exercise, pacing around a small room. Oh, we have a stationary bike we can put in your room, and you can use that as long as your platelet count isn't too low.

Ken suggests that the pathology slides might be ready, would I like to see them? I follow him downstairs again, we make our way through the lab, and he introduces me to a large, comfortable, and kindly-looking woman who strikes me as a prototype of a Norman Rockwell school nurse. She is the boss cytologist, been there for years, not an M.D., but an expert in cell morphology, probably better than most pathologists and clearly regarded as the final arbiter of the cell diagnosis on microscopic analysis of blood and bone marrow specimens. We move to a microscope with multiple viewing ports, fiddle with the eyepieces till we each have them in focus. We start with one of my original New

York Hospital slides. I haven't seen this before. The cytologist steers the slide around, focuses down on a nest of cells. Yes, myeloma all right, and look at those flame cells. Where? There, see the slight orange glow on the edge of those blue cells? Oh, yeah, like a burning match. Aggressive, cancerous, rapidly dividing plasma cells have that flame-cell appearance. There are a lot of them. I'm convinced, as if I wasn't before; there's nothing much to see but those monotonous blue cells. That's what the plasma cells of my myeloma look like.

Now for today's specimen. She loads it in, we peer again into our eyepieces. This is much better! She points out all the other cellular elements, growing white cells, red cells, platelet precursors, and, yes, still quite a few plasma cells, but not nearly so overwhelming. What do you think, how many? She hesitates. Well, we have to do a real count to be official, but . . . She squints into it again, years of experience clicking away in her head. I'd say it's about twenty-five, thirty percent. We look around some more, she steers the slide gently. Yeah, I'd say that's it. I don't know whether to feel sad there's so much or grateful there's enough to make contact with the antibodies on the special immunologic tests. Ken and I depart, and I notice that I'm not seasick. That's unusual. I always get a yucky carsick feeling when someone else is steering a slide around under a microscope and I'm just watching, it jerks my eyes around and somehow makes me feel sick. She must be a real expert—either that or I've never had such an interest in a slide before.

We head for the elevators, Ken wants to show me around the building. We go to the top floor, he has to drop some papers off, and I see a bunch of fancy administrative offices. Then we stop at the patient floors, which are on 12 and 14. No patient floor is ever called 13, even when it's the real thirteenth floor of a building. At New York Hospital there's 12 and 12A, so no one will know they are on 13, bad luck enough to be in the hospital. The fourteenth floor is a regular hospital floor, very modern, much like Memorial Hospital: the patient rooms, mostly semiprivate, all around the outside with views out the windows, and the nursing station and utility rooms in the inner, windowless core, centrally located to serve the periphery.

The twelfth floor houses the transplant unit at one end, with its own nursing station. All the attendants wear yellow gowns over their uniforms, most of them with masks on. All the rooms are single, and the doors have little glass windows. I peer in surreptitiously as I walk by, not wanting to disturb the patients' privacy, but curious nonetheless. A couple of doors have large glass windows, with patients staring out balefully. All the patients look the same, hospital gowns and robes, bald or wearing cotton turbans, not much facial hair, pale and yellowish skin, a uniform android look, I can't tell if they are men or women. Some are sitting in chairs reading, some are lying in bed staring at nothing. This does not look like a lot of fun, but no one I can see looks visibly distressed; it's a calm, relaxed atmosphere. Next to an empty room, I stop to read the sign taped to the door, which warns visitors to check in with the nurse first, hand in anything they want to bring into the room, and to scrub, mask, gown, and glove before they go inside.

Next to each room in the hallway is a large, slanted, waist-high table with large white sheets of paper ruled into squares. These are the flow sheets, where the minutiae of daily weight, urine output, IV inflow, food intake, lab results, medications, vital signs are recorded for all concerned to study before dealing with the patient. A quick look at this can tell the doctors and nurses how the patient is faring today, similar to the bedside notes in an intensive care unit. Yes, they appear to have a real system here, Anne did say they take very good care of patients.

How many transplant beds do you have? About seven, Ken says. This one here is the nicest one, we expanded into this room, which was originally a patient lounge. It is a large corner room, with window views in two directions, very sunny in late afternoon. I'll try to get this one for you, it'll give you more room to move around. That would be nice, I say, but someone might already have it. Well, we'll see, Ken says.

I get back to the number of beds. Seven isn't very many beds, and your turnover is pretty slow if most people are in for a month, isn't there a lot of competition for those beds among the transplant group? Well, yes, that's true, there is. So it could happen that I could get into remission and be ready to go, and then there would be a long waiting list. I don't think that would be a problem for you, because you would be the first patient with multiple myeloma to be treated, and that would take priority over patients we routinely treat for lymphoma or leukemia. Everyone would be very interested in seeing this new treatment regimen get started with a real patient. I feel relieved, but also a bit guilty that someone else might have to wait longer for his transplant because of me.

By now we're back in the clinic area. We walk by a tall, remote-looking man with sandy hair, glasses. Ken stops and introduces me to one of the big honchos Cox wanted me to meet. He had heard that I was coming up, is pleased to meet me. Ken explains I've been on the M2 protocol for a couple of months, am doing well, down to about twenty-five to thirty percent marrow involvement from over ninety-five percent, and we've been discussing modifications in that protocol. He smiles, says he's sure they could get me down to remission swiftly with something like VAD. I sense a certain disdain for the plebeian M2 regime. I also think about all the bad things VAD could do to me, don't like it one bit. I say we'll be talking to Anne Moore about it. We shake hands and Ken and I move off.

Ken and I go downstairs to his office. He pages Cox's good friend, who is more fully involved in actual clinical work with patients day to day and spends little time on lab research. Apparently Ken spends most of his time in basic science research, quite a lot of time every day running the blood component lab, and on the side he sees patients in the outpatient clinic and rotates with the other transplant team doctors as attending of the month, taking charge of the inpatients on the transplant service. Because Cox's friend, on the other hand, spends most of his time taking care of patients, Cox very much wants me to get this guy's perspective on bone marrow transplantation; first because he has more clinical experience than Ken, and second because Cox considers his friend to be a no-bullshit guy and figures he will give me the straightest possible story about transplantation. Cox's insistence on this has given me the idea that Cox has some reservations about the protocol.

Cox's friend is unavailable right now but will be down later. While we wait, Ken returns some phone calls and I leaf through a booklet of statistics on expected incidence from various diseases in 1986, and death rates of males and females of various causes. I note the expected number of multiple myeloma cases, 5000 women and 5000 men in 1986, I saw that before in the protocol. I spend a while browsing for causes of death, see that young people die more from violence than disease: accidents, homicides, suicides, especially common in men under thirty. I suddenly realize I am starved, no wonder, I missed lunch. How long has it been since I missed a meal? I can't remember. I've really been caught up in this today.

When Ken gets off the phone, I ask him what he knows about the poor prognosis of myeloma patients who respond extraordinarily well to chemotherapy, as reported to me by Bill Hamilton from some review article. We discuss this concept for a while and surmise that it could be that the tumors that are particularly aggressive, multiply very fast, are more susceptible to chemotherapy because they take up the chemo more avidly, and are thus dispatched faster. I get it, I say, it's like that Wall Street saying, pigs get fat, but hogs get slaughtered. Yes. But it is a two-edged sword; those cells still multiply rapidly, so relapse occurs swiftly, and with succeeding rounds of chemotherapy the tumor cells become more and more resistant to the chemo and eventually cannot be controlled.

That's the whole point of high-dose chemoradiotherapy, to finish off all the cells with a permanently lethal dose very early in the disease, before they become too well educated by low-dose chemotherapy. Bone marrow transplantation makes that possible. Certainly that makes sense to me. We have learned over the past generation that antibiotic therapy is much more effective in eradicating bacteria if given in high doses over a short period of time, rather than in low doses for prolonged periods.

Moreover, it has appeared that some of the more successful outcomes in the B-cell lymphoma patients who have been treated with autologous bone marrow transplants have been those whose tumors have been aggressive rather than indolent, because the cells seem to be more susceptible to the chemoradiotherapy.

Cox calls Ken to check if his friend has met with me yet, decides to join us. Soon after Cox arrives, his friend does, too. His office adjoins Ken's. Ken takes off for the riverboat volunteer shindig, promising to call me in New York by Friday with the results of the antibody testing of my marrow. Cox and I sit with his friend for a while and talk.

This guy is a small, wiry man with a thick shock of brown hair and a mustache, somewhat somber, probably my age. I ask him about getting lots of marrow at the harvest by going to other bones, I expand on my experience in fracture work, suggest that orthopaedic technology could help them harvest more marrow. He says that wouldn't work because of blood loss; when they suck the marrow out of the pelvic bones with the syringes, they of course are siphoning off a lot of blood as well, because the blood circulates freely in the marrow, and a large part of the volume they remove is regular blood. Later they separate the blood from the cells they need for the transplant and give back the red blood cells the night of the transplant, so the patient doesn't need too many transfusions. Basically they take as much as they can, which does involve several units of blood loss, but they want to stop before the immediate blood loss requires them to transfuse blood during the harvest, because they don't want to harvest and treat donated blood. After the harvest they make up for the blood loss as needed until the patient's own red blood cells are ready to be given back that night. To do what I suggest would involve massive blood loss, ten or twenty units perhaps, and would be too dangerous. Well, so much for that bright idea.

I raise the topic of deaths due to transplants in the lymphoma patients they've treated in a similar way. What about the guy with the liver necrosis, was that totally unpredictable? They're not sure, it came out of the blue, he was the only one who died of that complication in all the many transplants done here, both autologous and the sibling kind. Retrospectively, they suspect it may have had something to do with his having been a big boozer, bigger than they had thought; in fact, he had been drinking in the hospital. After that experience, they strongly recommend that patients consume no alcohol in the hospital. I am incredulous. You mean I would have to stop drinking? Yes. He is impassive, flat. I realize I had pictured myself sitting in a chair, watching TV and drinking beer, just as I do at home every night now, watching the Mets play. It seems like a terrible sacrifice, going on the wagon. Furthermore, he adds, it would not be a good idea to drink much at all the few days before you come in. I guess he thinks I'd tie one on. He may be right.

He starts talking about how I must give serious thought to the timing of the transplant, and whether it would be something that was right for me to undertake at this time, because it is a big deal. I stare at him blankly, realize he is suggesting I defer this treatment. What alternative does he think I have? You mean just keep going with chemotherapy that doesn't cure, just to keep going? Well, everybody's situation in life is different, and some patients have jobs they need to support their families, some people have young children they don't want to leave, and the risk is there that it might not work. You know, most of the patients we have treated so far are being treated for disease that has relapsed once, twice, even three or more times. They have had a lot of disappointments, sometimes they just don't want to risk another big disappointment. I think about this and find it hard to identify with. At least I don't have young children at home, that would be very traumatic, to leave preschoolers. My job will be hard to leave, but it would only be temporary, and my partners can cover for me while I'm gone.

Does this treatment make you lose your hair? Well, most patients have lost their hair already by the time they come into the transplant program, from the treatment that gets them ready for it, but they experience more hair loss from the radiation, and they usually lose all their body hair. For some reason, more is lost in the upper body than the lower extremities. I picture myself bald as a billiard ball, with hair on my toes. Eyebrows and eyelashes, too? That's variable, most people keep some.

He continues, Most people lose weight, about ten percent body weight is the average loss. I calculate. Seventeen pounds, hey, this program isn't all bad! In fact, he goes on, we recommend that some people deliberately gain weight before they come in because they can't afford the weight loss. I smile, that's hardly the case for me. I wonder if I'd lose fat or muscle; I guess that depends on whether I eat any protein. If I don't eat protein, I'd cannibalize my own muscle tissue.

How long do you think I'd be unable to work? He is dogmatic, You should stay out six months. Six months! I had been thinking maybe six weeks, eight at the outside. Why so long? It takes a long time to recover from this, and your immune system is slow to recover completely. You should not be exposed to the hospital and sick patients. But I don't take care of sick people, all my patients are healthy, are undergoing elective surgery, and the operating rooms are very clean environments. He is an implacable wall. You really should stay away from it. Also from crowds, restaurants, theaters, places like that, for several months. Also small children, although some of our patients have small children and can't avoid contact with them. I don't argue with him, but think to myself that if some patients go back to their small children at home, I could certainly go back to contact with my healthy patients in the office.

Speaking of restaurants, Cox and I realize it is getting late, going on seven. We have to get to dinner before my flight back to New York. I thank Cox's friend for taking the time to talk with me, and Cox and I go to his office, where Karen has just arrived.

Through dinner I tell them enthusiastically about all I've learned today. They are interested but seem reticent about sharing my enthusiasm. Cox tells me about his very good friend at Memorial in New York, the one who's been trying to recruit him to move his lab to New York, and gives me his home phone number, urges me to discuss this with him. I tell Cox I am reluctant to get involved with someone else, I trust Anne, and I'll discuss it with her. Cox says he hears she's very good, he's been checking her out; evidently she passed the test, because he's not suggesting I change doctors.

After our hasty dinner, Karen and Cox drive me to the airport, I just make the flight. Exhausted, I sleep on the way home.

When I get in the apartment close to eleven, Jim calls out, How was it? I walk into the bedroom, smile at him. Dana-Farber is the Rolls-Royce of cancer treatment hospitals. Jim perks up, this is the happiest he's seen me in a long time, and he reflects my enthusiasm with avid interest. I recount my day, all I've learned about the transplant, my sense that Ken is a good guy, that I can trust him. I dig into my briefcase and pull out the protocol, Here, you gotta read this. I interrupt his reading to say, I just hope I can get into remission so I can do it. Jim reaches over and squeezes my hands, gives me a wry, determined grin. You will.

THURSDAY, AUGUST 14, 1986

While I'm seeing patients in the office, my brother calls me. I think I just blew it, and I'm sorry, it just came out, that's all. What happened? He was talking with my older half sister about who was going to arrive when for our nephew's wedding next week and mentioned the gathering of all my full siblings and my parents for the blood test, to see if there is a tissue match for me in case I need a transplant. It was the first she heard about you. Oh, shit, I was going to tell her myself after the wedding, I didn't want to distract her with this problem this summer, when she had so much on her mind. Well, again, I'm sorry. Okay, I better call her.

The line is busy. I dial my mother. Her line is busy. They are talking to each other. I dial the unlisted number my parents use, and my mother answers. Oh, hi, guess who's on the other line? I figured she was, tell her to hang up so I can call her.

Ginny picks up on the first ring. Cesca! What do you think families are for? I am so sorry, so sorry you are going through this. I struggle not to cry, I've closed my door, but people walk in pretty indiscriminately. Well, I'm not very happy about it either, but things are looking up. I tell her a bit about my good response to chemo, about the possibility of the bone marrow transplant. The tissue-typing blood tests are just for backup, we really don't want sibling marrow, but it will be useful to know if I have a match with one of my four full siblings. Half siblings like her are only a half match at best. We make plans to have dinner together next week, on Tuesday, all four of us.

I go on with my office hours and think about the future. Suddenly there is some structure out there, a goal. The bone marrow transplant is a definite goal, and maybe even the end of my treatment, if it's not the end of me. I feel incredibly relieved that maybe there will be an end to this ordeal. I have not liked the vague, open-ended prospect of chemotherapy every five weeks for the foreseeable future, nor the possible danger of getting another bone marrow cancer, like leukemia, from prolonged chemotherapy.

Now that there is a game plan, I think I better tell the three other partners. Drew was right before when he suggested not telling them anything, particularly when we had no idea what was going to happen, whether I'd get better or not do so well. But now I have a timetable: it'll take a couple of months to get ready for this by getting into remission, then two or three months out of the practice. I have totally dismissed the six-month concept, no way I'll stay out six months. The other partners need to know I'll be out of the practice for a couple of months, and I resolve to tell them as soon as possible.

I start with Charlie Goodwin; he and I tend to have the latest office hours on Thursday, and at the end of the day I suggest that we go decompress with some beers at the bar down the street. We descend into the large room below street level. It's filling up already, the only space is at the very end of the bar near the beat-up jukebox blaring old Irish favorites.

We get our beers and Charlie starts to talk about his week, but I interrupt him, say I have something important to tell him, and it's a secret, he must tell no one, not even his wife. I have myeloma, Charlie. He fastens his bright blue eyes on mine as if I were telling him a joke. You're kidding. No, I wish I were, it's true, I've been on chemotherapy for about three months. Who else knows? Just Drew, Bill, and Fiske, and my immediate family. I explain that I've been keeping a lid on it at the office and want to continue to keep it a secret, but in the next few months I'll have to leave the practice for a while to get a bone marrow transplant. Charlie stares at me, still stunned, almost speechless, a rarity for Charlie, and I look around the bar, at the bare tables, plastic-covered chairs, dirty floor, a strange place to be discussing this, I suppose, but I feel comfortably anonymous here.

I fill him in on more details, but we soon digress to more beers and remembrances of the times we spent together studying for the boards, and celebrating passing. Charlie is still stunned, shakes his head often, states his disbelief. He offers to take my call anytime; if ever I'm not feeling up to it, he'll take over at the last minute. Thanks, but so far it's not a problem, and there will be plenty of call when I have to leave. Does my father know? Charlie asks. Did you tell him when he did your will? No, I haven't told him, he doesn't need to know, he just did the will. As we leave the bar, I tell him to wait before he mentions this to the two remaining partners, I plan to talk to them next week.

FRIDAY, AUGUST 15, 1986

After my early morning session with the residents, I go to my office, which is deserted, no one will be in till nine. I warm up the Xerox machine, copy all the Dana-Farber material for Anne, put it in a large manila envelope. I'll take it over to her later, along with the slides from my bone marrow, she's very interested in what it looks like now. I have errands to do this morning, and Jim wanted to get some work done in the office, so I'll pick him up around lunchtime and on the way home he can watch the car and I can deliver the packet upstairs at Anne's office.

I run into Anne herself on her way to lunch and we decide to have lunch together if it's okay with Jim. I lean into the car to ask him if he minds. Jim smiles, he knows it will mean a lot to me to have a chance to talk to Anne at length about the transplant. He drives off, and Anne and I go to the hospital cafeteria, settle at a secluded table in the back room where the faculty sits, a dim, dreary room with old murals that must have been painted in the thirties and never since refurbished, but with a clubby atmosphere nonetheless. Looking around the room I see the same faces that were there years ago when I had lunch with Anne when I was a lowly medical student, trespassing into this faculty preserve.

I tell Anne all about my day at Dana-Farber. I knew you'd like it, Cesca, they are very nice up there. I mention upping the chemo. Anne is cautious, warns me that the downside is I could get sick, have to be hospitalized for fever. It is a sobering thought. I decide to let her decide how much is enough.

We spend the rest of the lunch talking about our children, relaxing and having a good time together, like old times. We really have a lot in common, and we enjoy dropping the doctor-patient bit and being just friends again.

MONDAY, AUGUST 18, 1986

Ken Anderson calls me in the office. Good news, the antibodies attached to the appropriate cells in my marrow, so that's the major eligibility requirement of the protocol met. It's about 28 percent plasma cells on this test, which corresponds to the 25 percent on the bone marrow biopsy, the more traditional test. I tell Ken I'm still very enthusiastic about doing this, how soon does he think we can start? Well, first you have to be in remission. Yes, I know that, but how long do you think that will take. Oh, maybe a couple of months. Do you think we could do it faster if I had more chemo, bigger doses? Yes, but you should talk to Anne about that. I did, and she's cautious about moving up too fast, she doesn't want me to get sick. Also I gave her a copy of the protocol, is that okay, you don't mind? No, that's fine. Okay, well, thanks for calling, and I'll keep you posted.

I pass by my partner, George Zambetti, in the kitchen area of the office, standing room only by the ever present coffee machine. I ask him to come talk to me, if he has a minute. He follows me into my office and I close the door. George is five years younger than I and has been in the practice three years longer. He is a gentle giant of a man, a former Fordham basketball star, he can walk through the doorways of our office without ducking with at least a half inch of headroom to spare. He sits quietly, waits for me to start. He is not given to idle chitchat. I get right to the point, tell him about the illness, the proposed treatment. He is impassive, and stunned. He wonders if there is anything he can do for me. I cringe at that, the standard offer to a dying patient, but I say no, there is nothing to do, except keep it quiet, and not to even tell his wife. George stares out the window, remarks that it is always a surprise when something terrible happens, and we both know he is reliving the stillbirth of a baby he and his wife suffered a couple of years ago. We share a companionable sadness, a feeling of utter helplessness. There is little to say. I get up, head to the door to resume seeing my patients, and tell him all the partners know now except Jim Parkes, and I'll get to him this week if I can find him in one spot. George smiles, knows I am referring to Jim's well-known hyperkinesis; Jim is always flying by, offering a wave and a quick one-liner in passing, rarely stopping long enough for a conversation. As George gets up to go with a sad sigh, I tell him he can talk to me about this anytime, and I'll keep him informed as plans develop for my leaving for Boston.

TUESDAY, AUGUST 20, 1986

My partner, Jim Parkes, usually has office hours on Tuesday. I look for him after my surgery in the separate office he uses at the front of our building, facing Fifty-eighth Street. Amazingly, the waiting room is empty, and as I ask his secretary if he's in, he calls out to me to come right in. I enter his consulting room, close the door behind me, and peek into the examining room to make sure it's empty. I look at the walls plastered with framed photographs of baseball stars and other athletes he's treated, take a seat as he asks, How are you, dear? "Dear" is Jim's designation for all women, it always grates, but I realize it's habitual for him and let it pass, as usual. Not so hot, Jim, that's what I came to talk to you about. Mechanically, almost, I tell him of my diagnosis and proposed treatment, the time away from the practice. I am so sorry, he says, and for emphasis, repeats this two or three more times.

He relates the story of someone close to him who years ago had a bad tumor with a very poor prognosis, who has done well, no recurrence after many years, the importance of faith and hope. He tells me he and his wife stand ready to help me in any way they can. I appreciate that, but please don't mention this to her or anybody, it's a secret. He agrees to keep it quiet, stands with me as I leave to usher me out of the office. There, now all my partners know. I feel relieved.

FRIDAY AND SATURDAY,
AUGUST 22 AND 23, 1986

This is the weekend of my nephew's wedding, and my parents and all my siblings, who are coming to New York for the festivities anyway, have agreed to get their blood tested for the tissue typing. Anne had suggested this two months ago, before we knew about the autologous bone marrow transplant, when she was thinking of a sibling marrow transplant as an outside possibility for treating me aggressively. Now it looks as though that would be a more dangerous approach to take, compared to the Dana-Farber experimental technique.

But it will still be very useful to know if I have a sibling who matches me exactly in the tissue that creates problems in transplants, HLA, for human lymphocyte antigen, the special white blood cells that the immune system uses to tell if tissue is foreign or not. When the HLA matches, one is less apt to suffer rejection or graft-versus-host disease. If I ever have trouble with rejecting platelet transfusions from unrelated donors, I might do better with an exactly matched or closely matched sibling's platelets, so it's still worth doing.

Anne has everything organized, and we are all assembled in her office at 8 o'clock, way before regular office hours, because Memorial's lab has made a special concession to do this on a Friday instead of in the middle of the week, as they have to run the tests all day, even into the evening, if we don't get the blood to them early. Everyone is there on time. I am amazed, because my mother and Mimi are never on time for anything. The atmosphere is subdued, almost funereal. I sense my parents, my three brothers, and my sister are overwhelmingly aware of the seriousness of my illness and have a grim conviction that they want to help in any way they can. Daddy has not traveled to New York for years, and here he is to give a blood sample, witness to the gravity of the day. I have brought coffee, hand it around, trying to express, ineffectively, my gratitude that they are here for me. The blood drawing does not take long; when it's my turn, extra vials are taken for my routine tests and another protein electrophoresis.

MONDAY, AUGUST 25, 1986

I am struggling with writing up the paper I gave at the meeting in Vail in July. One of my friends is editing an issue of an orthopaedic journal that is to be entirely devoted to foot and ankle articles, and he asked me to write up my talk for publication. I blithely agreed to do it because I thought there would be nothing to it, but now I want to get out of it. I already called him last month after the journal sent me instructions for three copies of the paper, tables, and glossy black-and-white five-by-seven photographs of the illustrations with legends and everything, and a big bibliography. I just didn't feel up to it, especially assembling a big literature search, because I knew there wasn't anything in the literature to cite that was really relevant to what I was discussing. No problem, Francesca, you don't need a long bibliography, I really want your paper, I know it's going to be good.

So I've been struggling with it, got the slides made into prints, did cut-and-paste with my slide texts and a Xerox machine to assemble tables, found the few references and assembled them alphabetically for the bibliography. But my new word processing package is not working well for me because it's not like the old one on the old computer, and I just don't want to do it anymore.

I call my friend again, tell him it's not going well, in fact, it's a pretty stupid article. Besides, I'm sick, I wish I could tell him, and I don't want to hassle this. I know he knows I'm trying to weasel out of my agreement, and he won't let me. I say that I know it's the deadline already, and the paper is not done. That's okay, he says take a few more weeks, I know it's going to be very good. Okay. We hang up. Shit, I couldn't get out of it, could not use my illness as an excuse, because I don't want anyone to know, yet I know I'm having trouble with this paper because it's hard to mobilize the energy for anything right now, particularly anything that requires thought. So I plow on, finally figure out how to make this machine act like a typewriter, and whack it out some more.

THURSDAY, AUGUST 28, 1986

Today we are taking Heather to college, by plane. Kenyon College, in Ohio, sits on top of a hill, a graceful campus of stone buildings that seems timeless, shaded by stately trees and lined by straight gravel paths. At Heather's dorm we are greeted by friendly upperclassmen whose job is to carry the arrivals' belongings to their rooms. These guys are goodlooking hunks, enthusiastically muscling trunks and boxes up narrow stairways and around corners. Parents are greeted politely, but they seem to focus their attention on the new girls. I conclude the college has no trouble recruiting these volunteers, what better way to check out the arriving talent? Smith was not like this.

The afternoon's program is devised to achieve a deft

separation of parents from child. A convocation, an out-door reception, a group meeting with the faculty advisor, then the child is committed to meetings through the early evening so the parents might as well leave.

My separation qualms grow as the day goes on. I am reluctant to leave Heather here, worried about the bigger separation to come, who knows when, during the bone marrow transplant, wonder who will be there to support her if I get very sick, or worse. We chat with her faculty advisor and other parents. He is in the history department, a lean, blond man who is talking, for some reason, about his father's disappointment that he stayed in academics instead of coming home to run the chicken farm after college. I consider pulling him aside to ask him to look out for Heather because of my illness. I can't do it, sense that my emotional stability is too precarious to discuss this problem with the rebel son of a chicken farmer. Instead I tell Heather that she can share the secret of my illness with her advisor if she wishes. Okay, Mom.

We buy some beer, go to Heather's room, sit for a while and talk with her and her roommate as they unpack haphazardly. They have a dorm meeting before dinner, so we hug good-bye and go. On balance, it has been a comforting day. Jim loves the school, had not seen it before, and has the same impression I had when I toured Kenyon with Heather a year ago. We'd both love to be here as students, envy Heather for being in a place where time has stopped, the ivory tower, a good place to find yourself, grow up.

Tomorrow is our twenty-second anniversary, and we celebrate in the fanciest restaurant we can find in nearby Newark, Ohio. Our mood is nostalgic, we talk about times when the children were little, how did they get so big so fast? We hold hands and reminisce about our early years together, before children, echo each other's amazement that we lasted so long considering our difficulty in resolving disagreements, week-long sulks until we each learned not to expect the other to be a mind reader. Somehow we evolved together. I was really lucky to find you. No, I was the lucky one, Jim says. Okay, we were both lucky. We smile at each other, content and smug. I wall off thoughts about how little time we have left together.

TUESDAY, SEPTEMBER 2, 1986

Jim comes home from work sad and defeated. Things have been in turmoil at his company, which merged a year ago with another advertising agency, and the fallout continues as departments in the previously independent agencies jockey for power. Although he has been reassured that his talents are valued and they want him there, what is actually happening is a gradual erosion of his responsibilities. Another one of his jobs was lateraled to someone else from the other side today. Everyone in his department is looking for another job but him.

Maybe you ought to look around, prepare a résumé. Jim looks at me balefully. He has been with this agency since college, never worked anyplace else, has created at least three different new careers there that have been productive for his agency and fascinating for him. A media expert who taught himself data processing, he has a unique niche there, and he is a genius at solving media problems with computer solutions, as only one who knows media work from the inside could.

No, I have to stay, he says, for a lot of reasons. It isn't

just that he doesn't want to leave, that he doubts the availability of a comparable job elsewhere. We need his benefits. My only health insurance is through him. He doesn't want to rock the boat. I figure the bone marrow transplant may cost a hundred thousand dollars. We are still waiting to find out if his agency, which is self-insured, will cover the transplant. That's what major medical insurance is for, medical disasters. It has occurred to me, though, that they might figure out that they'd save a lot of money if they let Jim go. I wonder if coverage would be transferable if he left, but he doesn't want to ask, raise any suspicion that he may leave. I am no longer insurable on my own. But it must be against the law, or something, to drop someone's coverage when they get an expensive disease. It must be, and I am not sure.

If I weren't sick and facing the prospect of huge medical bills, the possibility of being unable to work, maybe even dying, Jim would have the freedom to leave this horrendous job situation. How can he stand it? I would find it intolerable. I would get out. He won't. I am both amazed and angry at his passivity, his resigned acceptance, his implacable, resolute staying-put. My guilt is enormous; if it weren't for me, he could find gratifying work, he is sticking it out for me.

The worst-case scenario grips me: I die, and Jim loses his job, how much can a guy take? I feel pretty helpless, very sad. Bone-deep dread grips me, and I stifle urgings to get out and get going on finding something else. I can't shore us up, he's probably right to stand pat, tough it out, but at what cost to him? Let's have a beer and watch the Mets game.

THURSDAY, SEPTEMBER 4, 1986

My complete blood count yesterday was totally normal. My hematocrit is up to a new high of 41, so my anemia has been corrected by the chemotherapy, even though I still, of course, have myeloma cells in my marrow; at least they aren't crowding out the red blood cells anymore. We are dropping the BCNU from today's chemo, and Anne is increasing the Cytoxan by fifty percent, to 1200 milligrams IV, and the Alkeran to 10 milligrams a day for a week, up from 8 milligrams a day. The prednisone will stay the same, 60 milligrams a day for a week, and a quick taper to none over three days. The vincristine will stay the same as before, too.

You sure this is enough, Anne, we can't push it a little more? We have lots of time, Cesca, you don't want to get sick. You don't have to rush into the transplant, they'll still be there when you're ready, don't worry about that. Let's see how you do with this dose, and we can try a little more next time. Okay, it's just that I want this to be over. Well, you're making great progress, the last IgG level from two weeks ago was down to 2400, a big drop from 3600 a month before. I wonder how long it's going to take. I don't know, but you're doing fine.

Back in the office that afternoon I get the bright idea that I could calculate a graph that would project how long it will take to get me in remission as Ken has defined it, less than five percent plasma cells in my marrow, no matter what the other lab tests show. Between patients, I scratch out computations by hand. Let's see, now . . . if I started with 95 percent tumor cells in my marrow and had 30 percent after three cycles of chemo, how much is the kill rate per cycle of chemo? Math has never been my strong point. We have to assume a linear rate. I try some multiplications of percentages against the percent of tumor cells in sequences of three, find that 66 percent works, accurately predicts that starting with 95 percent tumor cells, if the tumor cells left after a slug of chemo is 66 percent of what was there before, I have 28 percent tumor cells after three slugs of chemo, which is what it was. Good.

Now how does that project forward in time? Let's see . . . the fourth chemo will get me down to 18 percent, that'll be in early October, chemo number five will get me to 12 percent by early November, chemo number six will have me at 8 percent by early to mid-December, and I won't be close to remission till mid-January, when I'd be at about 5 percent tumor cells left. Shit, this is going to take forever. I look at the numbers, am amazed that the progress slows down so much as the percent of tumor cells get smaller.

Bill Hamilton drops in while I'm gazing at these numbers in consternation. I tell him what I've just figured out. Sure, he says, it's like taking half the distance to the door with a step, and he steps towards the door, then another one, again half the distance, smiles at me, says, You get closer, but you never get there. I get it. That's the problem with chemotherapy, the final step through the door.

Now I have a time frame. I'll be able to go skiing in Vail at the meeting we've been going to for the last few years, the second week in December, a wonderful time to be in Vail, no crowds, good snow, great restaurants. I'll be home for Christmas with the children, good. But the Academy of Orthopaedic Surgeons is meeting in San Francisco in January, and this is the year I'll be inducted as a fellow, the final ritual of acceptance into this profession, which I've been working toward for so long. Will I have to miss this? After years of striving? How unfair! I picture myself in the hospital while Charlie Goodwin and my other friends are there at the induction ceremony and feel very sorry for myself.

What else will I miss? We usually go to Italy in March to ski; in fact, I had been hoping Anne Moore and her family would join us in our house there; she was enthusiastic about it when we discussed it earlier this summer. I might miss this, unless I can start the transplant in early January. If I could start then, maybe I'd be out by mid-February, and could go to Italy by mid-March. We'll see.

I go down the hall at the end of the day to where Charlie Goodwin is finishing up for the day. I tell him about the high probability that I'll miss the meeting in San Francisco. Charlie is adamant, I want you to be there with me, Francesca. I agree, I want to be there, too, but it might not work out. But we have been through all that crap with the boards together, it won't be right if you're not there with me. He fixes me with his blue stare. I pull my eyes away to the window. That's the breaks, I say, but maybe it'll work out somehow. I think to myself, Whenever I go, I'll miss something important, but getting rid of this disease is the most important thing, that's the thing to keep sight of.

MONDAY, SEPTEMBER 8, 1986

I walk to the office now. I figure it's two miles across Ninetieth Street to the Engineer's Gate, down the park drive, across Seventy-second Street, and then a shortcut north of the Sheep Meadow to exit Central Park at Columbus Circle, a block or two from my office or Roosevelt Hospital. It takes about forty or forty-five minutes, if I walk briskly, and I do, plugged into my Walkman, listening to bouncy music. The problem with walking is it gives me time to think, and I can't shake my depression, despite the upbeat blast in my ears. The backpack housing my office shoes and handbag bangs against my back, slick with sweat, and I avoid the eyes of joggers heading uptown, don't want them to notice the tears slipping down my cheeks. I settle down by the time I get to the Sheep Meadow, brilliant green in the early morning sun, concentrate on the day ahead.

This morning I have a couple of patients in the office, then I'm doing a case together with a plastic surgeon. I referred this patient to her, he has a vascular tumor in his second toe, and she is experienced in vascular replantation of digits and microsurgery, should that be necessary in this case. I will help with the ankle anesthesia and the various approaches to the foot. When I get to the hospital I find out that the cases ahead of us in the operating room that we're supposed to start in at eleven are hopelessly long, and it will be at least one o'clock before we can get the case started. Great. There goes the day. Ruth will have to reschedule this afternoon's office patients till later, and I'll just be sitting around, waiting to go to the OR, sometime.

I go over to the office to see the two quick patients scheduled for ten. When I finish, I go into the consulting room I use on Mondays. It's Fiske's regular room, and Charlie Goodwin is schmoozing with Fiske. I collapse on the sofa and join in. After a while, Charlie leaves to see his patients, closes the door as he leaves.

Fiske asks me how it's going. I look away, stare out the window, speechless for a few moments, as I realize that how it's going is I feel like having a temper tantrum, two-year-old style. I want to throw things, scream and cry, bang my fists on the floor, throw a real purple snit. I'm losing it, Fiske, really losing it. He looks at my typed schedule on the desk, What're you doing today? Nothing this morning, my case is on terminal hold. Let's go for a walk, get out of here. Okay, let's.

We head toward Central Park, Fiske loping along with his duck-footed walk, just like Jim's, blue blazer flapping in the brisk air. I lengthen my stride to keep up. We slow up when we get to the baseball fields just south of the Sheep Meadow. We start talking about the Mets, the pennant race, still not clinched, individual players and their personalities. Ray Knight's intensity, he's not just wired, like Gary Carter, it's like he's receiving on all channels, a human satellite disc. We laugh, and I begin to lighten up.

We wander past the north side of the Sheep Meadow, head southeast into an area with tall shade trees and wide concrete walkways, benches on both sides. We settle down on a bench in front of a statue of a nineteenth-century notable. I lean back and look at the blue sky through an intricate mosaic of leaves, still green and dark against the sky.

I may be dying, I think, but there is sunshine here, and leaves, and stark branches, and blue sky. And a friend who's willing to hang out with my fear and weakness, my loss of spirit. No false reassurances that everything's going to be all right.

After a long, companionable silence, I say, I've been thinking maybe I should see a shrink. Oh, yeah? I've been so depressed. Trouble sleeping? No, no vegetative signs like that, or loss of appetite either, I say, laughing. I'm just so sad. I think I'd be angry. Yes, people say depression is just anger turned against the self—I am angry, but what I usually do when I'm angry is get depressed and cry. There's just no place to put it, no one to be mad at, no one I can blame.

More silence. There's probably not much point in seeing a shrink, anyway, it wouldn't take a rocket scientist to figure out why I'm depressed. I guess not. I saw a shrink for a while many years ago, I go on, it was very helpful. Oh? What was that about? Anxiety and depression when I was in medical school, I thought I was a lousy mother, I don't know. But I learned a lot and haven't had any trouble till now. But this is different, who wouldn't be depressed? It helps to talk about it. Fiske smiles, and this is a lot cheaper.

I look up at the leaves again, think about what the issues would be if I went to a shrink now. I don't know, but I don't think I want to get into it, there's always some ungluing that has to be done before you can put things back together, and right now my hold on my life is so tenuous, I don't want to risk letting it all crash down around me. Who would I go to? My old shrink knows me well, in fact I saw him at a large party last June, soon after my diagnosis. Jim and I chatted with him for a while, caught him up with the last ten years, all the doings except the essential new fact. I don't think he's into psychotherapy for the dying. He's more psychoanalytic.

We sit quietly, watch homeless denizens of the park shuffle by, an occasional young mother striding purposely with umbrella stroller and toddler. I look up at the sky again, think it would be nice if I had some tie to a religious faith. It just isn't there.

We're going up to Bill's place at the end of the month, I say. That should be great, it's beautiful up there. You been there? Yeah, it's not that far from where we go in the summer, we've taken the kids climbing near Lake Placid, and my nephews have trained on the ski jumps there, awesome. I want to get some maps of hiking trails in the area, Jim likes to hike. Eastern Mountain Sports probably has some, Fiske says, it's nearby, and I'm looking for a running watch.

We head off toward the store. You go to church, Fiske? No, not really, but sometimes I go to mass with Michelle and the boys, it's relaxing and quite peaceful, actually. I consider that and think of a friend of mine who also goes to church every Sunday without fail, and I envy the strength they must derive from a conviction that there really is a God. I have no personal belief in God, or something out there, nor do I know there isn't, either. I feel a bit bereft in the spiritual department, as my mother has pointed out on numerous occasions, but even now, I can't pretend to something that isn't there for me.

The store has no suitable watch for Fiske, but they do have maps, and Fiske helps me select the right geographical location, Keene Valley and environs. We stroll back to the hospital amid lunchtime throngs on Columbus Avenue. Fiske veers off to the hospital. See you. Yeah, so long. I go to the office, refreshed and restored, glad to have a friend like Fiske.

SEPTEMBER 9–25, 1986

The housekeeper just isn't working out. So far she's lost one of Jim's polo shirts every week while doing the laundry, and they were new. The food is indifferent to lousy, and I hear from the man in the valet shop in the lobby where we get our shirts and dry cleaning done that she's bitching to him about being overworked and underpaid. I need this? I come home early one Friday, tell her thank you, here's next week's pay, please leave your keys. Now what do I do?

The solution occurs swiftly. The woman who does the heavy cleaning for us on weekends arrives while we're still there, and I tell her I fired the housekeeper, she didn't work out. She says I should have told her I was looking for someone, because she has a friend who needs a job. This woman lives in her housing project, they are good friends and belong to the same congregation. And she's a wonderful cook. She doesn't have a phone, but she'll have her call me.

The housekeeper prospect calls me the next day, arrives at the apartment early the following day. She's great, as cheerful as the last woman was dour, and her plumpness hints at her being a good cook. We hit it off well, and I hire her on the spot. The apartment glows when we come home, dinner is delicious every night, and no laundry gets lost. This is heaven. The only problem is thinking of what to eat every night. I dig out old recipes from *Redbook* magazine, label them Good Dinner #1 to #12, put them in see-through plastic envelopes, tell her to cycle through them. She does them very well.

I'm upping my exercise schedule. Stretching and sit-ups in the morning, increasing time on the cross-country machine, walk to work, walk back if I'm not too tired, or take a cab or get a ride from Fiske. Exercise is my outlet, a way to channel my rage, although the rage still overwhelms me, particularly in the morning when I'm on the floor, stretching. I just stop and cry, this is my crying time, with the morning sun pouring in, the music blasting, God help the neighbors. One particular song has caught my imagination, a mournful dirge. I am mesmerized by it, play it over and over as I cool down, shower, and dress. An orgy of self-pity, I know, but this song expresses how I feel.

On my way to work, I wrestle with myself, berate myself for being such a fucking bad sport. This is what I feel the worst about. I want to be a good sport about this, take it in stride, be noble and brave, cheerful and sanguine; instead I cry all the time when no one's watching, feel it's unfair, wonder why I, of all the other more deserving people, got singled out for this malicious fate.

I try to think positively, focus on getting ready for the transplant. The more I'm in shape, the better off I'll be. If my cardiac function is the best it can be, if I develop tremendous cardiopulmonary reserve, then if I get infected during the time of no white cells, maybe I can withstand septic shock. This has got to be good for me, all this exercise. Also, it's a well-known fact that aerobic exercise releases endogenous endorphins, our very own feel-good, morphine-like, anti-depressant substances. I'm still waiting for this effect, but it probably takes time. All this exercise takes time, too, but getting ready for the transplant is like training for a marathon, I guess, and that's the best way for me to spend my time while I'm waiting.

J gets off to school. The apartment is quiet, and incredibly neat with both children gone. No more running shoes and other signs of adolescent life forms trailed around the living room in the morning when we get up. J's making an enthusiastic start at school. If he starts having problems I'll have to clue his class dean in to the troubles at home, meanwhile we'll let things ride and see how it goes.

Jim and I have started horseback riding on weekends. Riding was one of the great pleasures of my childhood, and I have been thinking about taking it up again for years but have somehow never gotten around to it. Now is the time, I may not have another chance. We go to the stables in Litchfield where my parents sent my horse and me to learn to jump.

It's no longer possible to rent horses by the hour and go out for a ride because the liability hazard is so great for the stable; we have to have lessons with an instructor, in the ring, till they get to know us. Ring riding was always boring, but we soon make it interesting by starting to take our horses over small jumps under the tutelage of the instructor. Jim is very good at this. He spent days on his pony as a child, has never had formal lessons, but he catches on very quickly. We graduate in a couple of weeks to the outside course, more fun in the wide open. Jumping is exciting for me, I enjoy a reckless abandon.

I'm feeling devil-may-care, start thinking about sky diving, talk about it to Bill, who shakes his head at me. No, really, Bill, what the hell? All these things like skydiving, surfing, scuba diving that used to scare me now seem like things I'd like to try. Why not?

The following weekend I nearly pitch off my horse when he refuses a jump, wrench a thigh muscle badly hanging on. A sobering experience. I picture an open fracture of both bones of my forearm, no, that wouldn't be so keen right now. I guess I won't go skydiving, I could break an ankle if I land wrong. The next day we get our instructor to take us out on the trails and dirt roads, this is really what I like, the gritty sound of horseshoes on gravel, the smell of dry leaves in the woods, the easy swinging gait of my horse beneath me.

My brother John calls me to say he and Joan are going to take an evening course in creating results in your life, would we like to join them? This would be a follow-up to the beginner course that Jim and I had done with John a year and a half ago, it was somewhat mannered, but it had useful exercises and tapes that helped me to focus on creating results I wanted to achieve. Back then it was passing the boards. Jim wants no part of it, ostensibly doesn't want to drop his piano lesson on Thursdays, but probably does not want to look at the issues of what he's got at work and home compared to what he wants. John and Joan will be there, and they'll have their car, so there will be no problem getting back from way downtown where the weekly evening meetings will be held. John urges me to do it, suggests that there may be some very big results I'd like to create. No shit, John. Okay, I'll do it. I call the woman who's running the course and sign up, the first meeting is October 2.

My blood count at the expected low point following the last chemo is quite high, the white count dropped to only 3.5, just barely under normal. I wonder if it was enough of a blast. We plan the next session for October 6.

The results of the tissue typing are back: I have no exact match with any of my siblings, just a half match with each of my three brothers and a total mismatch with my sister, no good for a marrow transplant. Good thing we aren't counting on a sibling transplant for my treatment. I tell John and Reto that they actually match each other exactly, which surprises them because they consider themselves to be quite different from each other, and John says he is not surprised that my sister and I are a total mismatch. In point of fact, however, this tissue typing relates only to genes that express antigens on white blood cells that would cause allergic reactions to transplanted tissues. The tissue typing has no relation to any genes involved with looks, or personality, or temperament. And if I ever get into trouble with platelet transfusions, my brothers are the closest tissue match I have.

By the middle of the month, several weeks after the deadline, the paper I had promised to my friend for the orthopaedic journal he is editing is written and ready to send off. I think it's terrible, but if my friend doesn't like it, he can edit it. At least I can put it out of my mind.

A few days before our planned weekend with Bill and Linda, Bill tells me Linda can't go, her job as a ballet dancer requires her to rehearse with the ballet company on Saturday, plus she has work to do in her psychology graduate courses. Bill is still enthusiastic about the trip, and we have both blocked out Monday so we can take a three-day weekend. I am hanging on for this weekend, really feel a need to get away and relax, getting through each day is more and more of a struggle to maintain composure, not fall apart. I am feeling very fragile.

By Wednesday, Jim decides he doesn't want to go. Linda won't be there, he says, the five-day weather forecast is bad, so hiking will be out, and I'd have to miss the Giants game on Sunday traveling down by train instead of by car with Linda as planned. Plus I have a load of work to catch up on at the office. You go, it's okay, have a good time. Are you sure? Yes, please go, you and Bill will have fun together, and I know you've been looking forward to it for a long time.

I find Bill in the office, ask him if it would compromise his reputation totally in Keene Valley if I came up for the weekend without Jim. Bill chuckles. My reputation was ruined long ago, Francesca, don't worry about that. We'll have a fine time. We decide to leave midafternoon on Friday from the office.

WEEKEND, SEPTEMBER 26–29, 1986

Bill and I head up to the George Washington Bridge in plenty of time to miss the worst traffic. The weather is clear, brisk and gorgeous. I pull out some tapes, start one that I tell Bill is a collection of my favorites. As Bill listens, he exclaims in amazement, I didn't know you liked C and W! C and W? Country and western, he explains. I grin. Well, it's one of my lowbrow secrets. Bill says he was raised on this music in Oklahoma and Tennessee, still loves it. He paws through his beat-up L. L. Bean bag, which houses an enormous collection of tapes, selects some old country classics he has taped from his record collection, and we listen raptly as we hurtle up the thruway. The colors change as we head north, just a few hints of real color emerge as darkness falls. By the time we get to the scenic route north of Lake George it is pitch-black out, and I wonder how the color really is up here, hope we're not too early for it.

Bill's house is a cozy, rebuilt cabin, green clapboard on the outside, modern on the inside, the central area dominated by a huge stone two-story fireplace emerging from a pit of built-in sofas, chintz pillows, and pineboard walls. I'm using the sleeping loft, where the bed hangs from the ceiling on four ropes, and swings when I sit on it. I hope I don't get seasick.

The house is cold. Bill turns up the heat, and we go to grab a late dinner at a German restaurant some miles away. We have a pleasant time, chat about our lives before medical school. Both of us had been grown-ups for a number of years, he in engineering and business, army in Germany, me in social work and raising children, before we turned our lives around and reentered the adolescence of medical education. Funny how such disparate backgrounds wound up in the same field, partners in the same practice, and, moreover, sharing a special interest in foot and ankle problems.

In the morning Bill plays golf with a couple of friends, and I go around with them, enjoying the fresh air and the exercise of walking from hole to hole. No, I don't play, I decline gracefully. I took golf for physical education at Smith, but all we ever did was hit a five-iron, and I'm probably the only one who sprained an ankle in golf class. I got a C minus, the worst grade on my transcript, and I would have failed without a doctor's note about the sprained ankle. No, thanks, anyway, I'll just walk around with you. The views are spectacular, green fairways bordered by woods blazing with reds and oranges. The leaves are on the course, too, and at this time of year bright orange golf balls are harder to spot. Bill's friends are friendly and pleasant, and if they think my presence is strange, they give no sign of it.

These two golfers are coming to dinner at Bill's tonight, and the wife of one of them is bringing the main course, a gumbo. Bill and I shop for the rest of the meal and then Bill takes me on a driving tour down the Au Sable Club's miles-long dirt road to some back lakes. It is gorgeous, perfect for riding or hiking. We climb a trail to a view of the lakes, quite a vertical climb, but I manage to keep up without too much breathlessness.

Bill has heated the hot tub on the second-story deck, which looks out on a lovely view of the valley, and we warm up in the hot water. I try a wine cooler, stay in the water till my submerged skin resembles corduroy, very relaxing. I am beginning to unwind. Bill makes the dessert, a cooked apple and brown sugar tart he learned from his mother, and I set the table in an effort to be useful. The guests arrive and we chat pleasantly about our children, after Bill and I respectively have called home and checked in with our absent spouses.

The gumbo and Bill's dessert are excellent. Everyone is groggy after dinner, and leaves soon, the men planning another golf game, weather permitting, this time at the Au Sable Club course.

Bill and I breakfast at the local diner, and then Bill introduces me to Lucifer, his Model-T Ford. Bill cranks up Lucifer, and we go for a little drive on back roads. Lucifer can't go very far, though, and Bill wants to show me White-face Mountain and Lake Placid, so we switch cars and drive over to the mountains. The weather is overcast, but I am still entranced by the color. I want to drink it all in, etch it indelibly in my soul. Sadness overtakes me again as morbid thoughts occupy my mind, thoughts that I may never see another fall, this is the last one, my last favorite time of year. And here I go, being a bad sport again. I sort of want to talk about it, but all I can say to Bill is that I'm having a hard time not feeling like a bad sport about things. I can tell I'm making him uneasy, he says it's pretty natural to feel that way, who wouldn't, and we continue our tour.

In the afternoon, while Bill is playing golf, I walk all the way up the dirt road we drove up yesterday, take a few side trails as well, and rejoin the men on the last few holes of the golf course. It was a wonderful walk, but I'm tired. I resolve to increase my exercise, start to run a bit; really, getting in shape is the most important thing, I could spend more time on it, maybe a couple of hours a day.

On Monday we have a lazy morning finishing the Sunday *Times,* then close down the house and head off to New York. After a rainy morning the sun is bright as we drive the eighty miles of scenic, undeveloped land north of Lake George, the foliage is really at its height. The traffic is light, and we make it into New York in daylight, spending the last couple of hours of the trip listening to the "Ode to Joy" chorale. It's been a wonderful weekend, and Bill has been the consummate host and friend, taking this whole weekend to show me a good time, cheering me out of my blues. I've really had a good time, and I think he has too.

OCTOBER 1986

The first session of the course I'm taking with John and Joan is Thursday night. In short order we are under way with a closed-eye exercise and are asked by the leader to imagine our own deaths. What is this?! I hang on tight, but this is ungluing me. We open our eyes. I am visibly upset and shaken, and John looks at me, he who has taken this course before, is reviewing it and persuaded me to sign up, John looks at me and says he is sorry, he had honestly forgotten this was the first thing we did, he would have warned me.

Now the leader opens the discussion to the group, and various members recount the insights they gained from this exercise. Joan puts her hand on my shoulder, urges me to talk about what's going on with me. I shake my head wordlessly, grasping for a little self-control. No, I can't talk about it, it's secret, yet I want to talk about it. I ask the group leader if this group is a safe place, is everyone agreed that what we talk about here is not repeated outside? She looks around at the group, everyone nods yes, certainly, it is a solemn agreement.

I start to talk. I am dying, I say, and that exercise is where I've been for some time now. I start crying too hard to talk, and everyone waits. Finally, I look up, and explain some more. I have a fatal disease, and there's a radical, dangerous treatment I'm going to have, a bone marrow transplant, and I want it to work, but I don't know that it will. I guess that's why I'm here, I have a big thing I want to do, I want to get a cure, but no one has ever been cured of this before. The group is silent, but I can see sympathy and support in their faces. I feel better for having voiced my doubts, realize that I have been afraid to embrace the concept of a cure, afraid that I would seem ridiculous to want so much, to state baldly that I intend to be the first person ever cured of this disease, afraid of deluding myself with false hope, magical thinking.

By the end of the first meeting, we have worked our way through various goals, and I have advanced from wanting a cure for my cancer to articulating my overall goal for this course, written in my notebook: I will be the first of many total cures of multiple myeloma.

*   *   *

I reread *The Path of Least Resistance,* by Robert Fritz, inventor of this seminar; I do my mental exercises, listen to the tapes daily. I don't know how it works, indeed it seems hokey to my medical mind, and yet it makes me feel better, gives me a chance to own up to my rage and helplessness and despair, to take the energy of those black emotions and rechannel them, to focus with light and clarity on my goal of getting ready for the transplant, both physically and mentally.

From time to time I realize I want to chuck it all, give up, turn my face to the wall and die. I let myself feel those thoughts, and then I focus on my goal again; hey, it's not just me, it's everyone with this disease in the future, this disease is beatable, it should be routine within ten years to be cured of this disease.

On Monday morning, October 6, I go to Anne's office for another bone marrow. This time we are shipping it by air express to Ken Anderson, so he can do the special antibody testing on it. This one hurts a lot more than the others; Anne says it's not unusual, the more you have the more they hurt. I can guess why: the bone heals the holes with callus, thick scarred bone, so it means there's more unanesthetized bone to bore through to get to the marrow. If my blood tests are okay today, we do chemo number five tomorrow. Before I leave, Anne insists that I get a flu shot, they've just come in, and it is highly recommended that people on chemo get this protection.

After surgery the next day I go over to Anne's office again. I did so well on the last cycle that we'll increase the Cytoxan from 1200 to 1400 milligrams, and the Alkeran from 10 milligrams a day to 12 milligrams a day for a week. We'll drop the vincristine. The prednisone stays the same, 60 milligrams a day for a week, then a rapid taper. I still have hair, but it's thinned in a way that's very noticeable to me. Maybe if I get it trimmed a bit it will curl more and cover the scalp that's peeking through.

I decide to go to a movie Jim doesn't want to see, it's nearby. I buy a ticket, and have a half hour to showtime. I decide to get a beer, Anne said hydration is important. I go to a nearby baseball bar, sit at the bar, and quaff two beers rapidly. The man next to me is smoking, and although I stopped over fourteen years ago, I really want a cigarette now. I bum one from my neighbor. I sit and smoke my cigarette, drink my beer, and reflect on how I'm soaking up the poisons, what the hell is beer and a cigarette in the face of chemo number five? I'm getting that reckless, I-think-I'll-take-up-skydiving feeling again. I finish my cigarette and go to the movie alone, something I have rarely done.

The bone marrow results are very good, down to maybe ten percent plasma cells, better than I expected. Ken and Anne are very encouraged, and so am I. Maybe the increased chemo has changed the slope of the curve I figured out before, assuming a linear rate. Maybe I'll be ready sooner than midwinter.

I reorganize my life to allow more time for exercise. I leave office clothes in my locker at the hospital so I can jog to the hospital in my sweats, then cool down and shower once I get there, saves a lot of time. Now that I've gotten over the episode of back pain, I figure I'm up to jogging, despite what Anne said months ago. I join a health club with a personal one-on-one trainer, so I have to do it, because you pay anyway if you cancel at the last minute, a good motivator. I do three sessions a week, and Drew switches early morning conference with me so I can teach the residents on Tuesday, go to the health club on Monday, Wednesday, and Friday early in the morning. I walk about an hour and a half a day, and jog or use the cross-country machine for twenty or thirty minutes on Tuesday, Thursday, and sometimes the weekend as well. Two hours plus a day isn't too much, this is the most important thing I can do to get ready, more important than anything else. When people at the hospital remark on my drenched sweatsuit, I smile and tell them I'm getting ready to ski in December.

The baseball season is coming to an incredible finish. The playoff series between the Mets and the Houston Astros is heart-stopping. I have identified with the Mets more strongly than ever, if they can do it, maybe I can do it. When I root for them, I root for me. The Wednesday afternoon game is depressing and unexciting at first, countless innings of no-score ball, with the Mets behind. I keep track of the game through office hours, and the game should have been over by the time I'm finished. The Mets tie it up, they go to extra innings. We are hooked into it. Bill has a Sony Watchman, and Fiske and I watch with him, no one able to leave because something might happen in the next few minutes. More scoreless innings, then the Mets lead, but the Astros tie it up again. Finally, in the sixteenth inning, the Mets win. It's exhilarating! If the Mets can do it, I can do it.

The World Series is agonizing, too. I get tickets to the second game from a friend at the hospital, the Mets lose. They're down two–zip. They win two out of three in Boston. Saturday night's game could decide it, and we have a long-standing dinner engagement in Litchfield, are being taken to a fancy restaurant for a dinner for eight, I can't just tell my brother, who is hosting this event, Sorry, I have to stay home and watch the World Series. Too rude. Instead I put a small transistor radio in my pocketbook and sneak off to the bathroom so often everyone is thinking I have a urinary tract infection, until I confess that actually I'm keeping an ear on the game. The game is far from over when we leave, and we listen through the static to the radio in my brother's car, and then watch at home as the Mets, down to their last out in the ninth inning, come from behind to tie the Series for a final playoff game at Shea. If the Mets can win, I can get a cure. They've pulled it out so far.

Fiske has a ticket for me to that final game. After the fourth inning, we meet a friend of Fiske's at the hot dog stand, an orthopaedic surgeon in Indiana who has flown all the way to New York to be at this game. He comes back to our box with us and shares my seat, not a problem at this point in the game, because no one is sitting. The Mets start a rally, the chant of the crowd is awesome, visceral, a solid wall of sound that reverberates in my chest like a drum. The Mets win! They win! If they can win, I can win!

My practice is busy, and I enjoy it, but I notice I'm pulling back a bit. I've cut my office hours shorter to leave me more time to exercise. I still enjoy my patients, feel a rapport with them. Fiske asks me how I can stand it, listening to what must seem like trivial complaints of tendinitis or heel pain when my problems are so much greater. No, it doesn't bother me, because I can understand how they feel. They are scared they have something really wrong and need some reassurance that the X ray is okay, they don't have a bad disease, their pain is pesky, perhaps, but not dangerous. In a sense, I reassure myself by reassuring them, or at least gratify myself through them in a way I cannot achieve for myself, yet.

My hair is really getting thin. Every time I comb it more hairs come out in the comb, every time I wash it, daily when I exercise, there are a few hairs in the drain, not much, but the effect is cumulative, and my once thick hair seems sparse, my scalp very noticeable. I better get a wig that matches my new hair color, my great idea about dyeing my hair to match the first wig really backfired and it would be very strange to change my color back to mousy from reddish. I go back to the same shop and buy another wig. It's much thicker than my own hair, even after we trim it, but it is the same color as my dyed hair, and the same style and length. I wear it back to the office on a quiet afternoon, hoping no one will notice. Fat chance. Fiske has a hard time controlling his amusement, and one of the secretaries notices it on her way out in the evening and asks me point-blank if I'm wearing a wig. No, no, I say, I just got it styled and it's all gunked with spray. This is not going to work, it's so damn obvious. I guess I'll stick with my own hair till there's none left.

NOVEMBER 1986

On November 10 it's time for another bone marrow. Actually, it's time for another chemo session as well, but I ask Anne to postpone it for the results of the marrow, just in case we're ready to move into high gear. Another very painful marrow is sent off to Ken in Boston. I don't hear from him as expected on Wednesday, and on Thursday I call him. He's very distressed. What's the matter? Well, it looks like the specimens are mixed up, or you have another disease. Another disease? What other disease? Something worse? Yes. You better talk to Anne, I tell him. I call Anne, then she hangs up to talk to Ken, who is calling. Anne calls back, I tell her I'm very alarmed. Relax, Cesca, your marrow is fine, I looked at it and it looks normal, they are just having trouble with their test, and they're confusing your regenerating marrow with something else. You mean I haven't all of a sudden developed leukemia too? No, of course not, just relax and let them work out their problems with their test.

I think for a while. If they are having trouble with this test, then we won't know if I'm ready for the transplant or not. Unless we do another marrow. I call Ken back. How about another marrow? I can fly up now, or tomorrow morning. No, it's too late now, and tomorrow I'll be away, I'd have to get someone else to do the marrow. That's okay, just tell me what time to be there. Okay, I'll call you back. The earlier, the better, I say. He calls back, nine A.M. in the adult clinic. Fine.

I tell Ruth to move my office hours back to noon. I should be able to make that. I take the early shuttle, a cab to the hospital, and after very little waiting Ken's substitute meets me in the clinic and we get another marrow. I thank him and he looks at me startled, says, I don't think anyone has ever thanked me for doing a marrow before. I laugh, Well, it is painful, especially a second one in a week, but I do appreciate your taking time out of your schedule to do this for someone who isn't even your patient. I grab a cab out on the street, make the 10:30 shuttle, and am back in the office just in time for office hours.

On Monday I go to Anne's office early for chemo number six. We haven't heard from Ken yet about the bone marrow, and I am still hoping that maybe I'll be ready now for the transplant. Anne voices caution, reminds me that there's plenty of time, I can wait and do other things, like be at home for Christmas. I can time the transplant so it's more convenient for me. I think about that, again, then say, But this is the most important thing, I've talked to Jim and the children about it, and Christmas isn't as important to any of us as my getting this over with, that would be the real Christmas we all want.

We decide to go ahead with the chemo, after I confirm with Anne that we could switch to the high-dose consolidation chemo right in midstream today or tomorrow,

187

because Cytoxan would be used, she could adjust the dose, and I can hold off on the Alkeran and prednisone till tomorrow. Anne's upping the dose to 1600 milligrams of Cytoxan from 1400 and 14 milligrams a day of Alkeran from 12, because again I've done well and the counts did not drop very low last month.

As Anne is hanging the IV Cytoxan the tube slips and some of the Cytoxan runs out on the floor. Oh, no! This is a problem, there's no way of telling how much ran out, so the whole batch has to be prepared again. Anne says the pharmacist can fix another dose, but it'll take about twenty minutes. That's okay, Anne, I have all morning. I read the paper and wait.

Anne walks in, saying, Guess who just called? Who? Ken, he says the bone marrow was perfect. Yeah? He says we can do the consolidation treatment. My mind whirls, I'm there! This is it. I feel relieved and scared at the same time. Anne looks at me, says, Well, Cesca, it's up to you, just remember, you don't have to do this now, you have plenty of time, you can wait. They will be there for you later if that's what you want. I consider that. No, I want to do it now, I want to get it behind me. Let's do it now.

What do we do? We'll give you 1200 milligrams of Cytoxan a day for four days. Do I have to be hospitalized? No, we used to hospitalize people for this much chemo, but now we can do it as outpatient treatment, but you must drink a lot of fluids to protect your bladder and report any burning on urination or bleeding so we can treat you right away. Okay.

I get out my diary book, we schedule the next three treatments. I look at my plans for the next month, count out the five weeks it usually takes for the marrow to recover from chemo, try to figure out when I'd be ready for the bone marrow harvest. The week of December 22. I wonder if they'll have a bed for me on the transplant unit. I look at early December. From the fifth of December through the seventh there's a foot and ankle course for orthopaedic surgeons here in New York, and I have to give a talk on Saturday the sixth. Then on the seventh we're flying to Vail for the winter Trauma Society meeting. It's going to be especially good this year because the group of us who were Roger Mann's fellows are going, and the whole meeting will be focused on foot and ankle problems. Bill Hamilton is going and will share a condominium with Jim and me. I hope I can go, I want to go, I should recover enough by then, let's see, that's a little less than three weeks from now.

Various dates and possibilities whirl through my head, I can't keep track of it all. One thing sticks, though: I'm leaving everything behind. Jim and the children can come with me over Christmas, but I have to leave my patients, my work, my friends, my partners, my family in Litchfield. Incredible sadness overwhelms me. I have to stop work, go away. How am I going to explain this? I can tell my patients I'm going on a sabbatical. But the other doctors at the hospital, all the doctors who refer patients to me, are going to think there's something fishy going on. People just don't up and leave a thriving practice to go on a sabbatical. They'll probably think I'm in the loony bin, or drying out someplace. I have to figure something out.

I call Jim from Anne's office and tell him the good news. He's thrilled, the waiting is over. I knew you could do it!

I go back to my office and see patients. I call Ken again, start negotiating a time for the harvest. They usually do the harvests on Tuesdays and Thursdays. Five weeks from now would be Christmas Day, how about the week before, the eighteenth, would that be too soon for the marrow to come back? No, probably not. Is the time booked yet? No, I don't think so. How about a bed on the transplant unit, will one be available then? I don't know, it's too soon to say who will be ready to leave, but I don't think you'll have to wait very long, we usually get a bed within a week or two of a harvest. I'm crestfallen. A week or two? Two weeks? We leave it that he'll pencil me in as a possible harvest for the eighteenth. I wonder if I'll be in the hospital on Christmas, or waiting for a bed.

Ken reminds me that there are tests that need to be done for the protocol, cardiac and pulmonary function tests, more blood tests. We plan for December 2; my counts should be coming back by then, I can easily make another day trip to Boston. He agrees to set up all the appointments. I tell Ruth to hold off on booking any surgery for December 2.

I tell my partners that it looks like it will be soon, maybe in the next five or six weeks. No, I don't know yet what I'm going to tell people, I'm still thinking about it. Bill asks if I've broken the news to Ruth yet. No, not yet, but I'm going to have to tell her soon. I can't face it, telling Ruth will be hard.

I think about the other women in the office, each partner's secretary, the office manager, the X-ray technician. I'm going to have to tell them too. I think I'd rather do it myself, face-to-face, so it's out in the open, no whispering behind my back, no unfounded rumors. The office is like an extended family, and I will need a united family behind me when I'm away, and each one of them deserves to hear from me personally, not through the office grapevine, that I'll be away, and why, and what we are going to tell patients. But I think I'll wait till just before I go into the hospital.

I get my second blast of Cytoxan on Tuesday, then I go to the hospital for my clinic, go to my committee meeting, and return to the hospital to see the woman I'm operating on the next morning. This is a snap, I'm feeling fine, a little head cold, but that's unrelated to the high-dose consolidation chemotherapy.

Everything changes in the evening. I feel wretched, nauseated, and by two A.M. I've thrown up so much there's nothing left but dry heaves. Compazine hasn't touched this terrible malaise. The high-dose chemo has caught up with me in spades. By morning I can barely stand up, and I realize there's no way I can operate today. I have never, ever, been too sick to operate, and now I'm too sick to stand in the kitchen to make coffee.

I call the operating room, tell them I have the flu, and cancel my case. My head cold has worsened, so I sound pretty coldy, and my story is convincing to the OR supervisor. I call my patient and explain the situation to her as well, saying we'll have to postpone the operation, I'm too sick to do my best work on her, and she can hear how lousy I sound too.

I go back to bed, lie in the room in the dark with the blinds shut, and drift. Too sick to sleep, too sick to have any light in the room, much less radio or TV, this is the strangest thing I've ever experienced. Later in the morning I mobilize myself to call Ruth and tell her I have the flu, I can't make office hours today or tomorrow, I'm hoping by Friday I'll feel well enough for office hours in the afternoon.

In the afternoon I go to Anne's office for the third dose of Cytoxan. I'm feeling a little better, but I dread the effect of this next dose, and tomorrow's. I tell her of my terrible night, that Compazine didn't touch it, no help at all. I ask her about Marinol, I've read about it in a magazine article that came out recently on coping with chemotherapy. THC, the active ingredient in marijuana, has been purified and is available in pill form for cancer patients with nausea and vomiting and malaise from chemotherapy. Sure, you can try it, I'll give you a prescription. On my way home I pick it up, read the package insert. It says to take it before you feel bad, it works better that way than if you wait, because in pill form it takes an hour or two to work.

I take the Marinol, two round brown pills, when I get home. By the time Jim is home, a few hours later, I am mellow, giggly, and very stoned. No nausea, no vomiting. Of course, I can't do anything, either, because I'm so wigged out. No matter, this beats throwing up. I take another dose before I go to bed and get a good night's sleep.

With my little brown pills, I weather the fourth and last dose of Cytoxan uneventfully. Very uneventfully, because I'm so stoned I don't feel like doing anything. By Friday morning, though, my brain has cleared, I feel okay, and I go into the office to see a few patients.

It's time to tell Ruth what's going on. She's been juggling my schedule all week, and it's really going to be topsy-turvy now. I wait till everyone has left, then sit down with her and explain the whole scenario. Much to my amazement, Ruth is not undone, dissolved in tears, bereft. No, she's furious. That really sucks, she says, in a rage. Just when you have everything together after all those years of hard work, it's just not fair, it sucks! This is a side of Ruth I haven't seen in the four years she's worked for me, and I'm a little nonplussed. We get down to business. I reassure her that she will still work for me, that we need her to manage my practice while I'm away; she knows my patients, and will direct them to Dr. Hamilton and Dr. Patterson for follow-up. We will tell my patients I'm going on sabbatical. Meanwhile, this is still a secret. I will talk to the other women in the office before I go, but she can tell her husband in confidence if she wants.

After a restful weekend, I feel fine on Monday, see a full schedule of patients. One is a man who wants his problem corrected surgically over Christmas, or soon after. I tell him that I'm probably leaving on a sabbatical about then, and he'll have to decide if he wants to wait till I get back or see my partner, so he can do the surgery. He decides to see my partner, and I direct him to Bill's secretary to make an appointment. He thanks me, and on his way out, calls out, Enjoy your sabbatical. I get curious looks from the secretaries who overheard. You're going on a sabbatical? Maybe, I say, and quickly call another patient in to avoid further discussion.

Surgery goes well on Tuesday. I'm feeling fine, and still walk back and forth to the hospital, although I've stopped the rigorous workouts.

On Wednesday morning I see Anne, get my blood checked. The white count should be showing a dip now. Anne calls me in the afternoon. Cesca, I can't believe you're in the office seeing patients. I feel fine, Anne. Well, your white cells are under 1000, 900 to be exact, you ought to go home and stay there. Don't go to Litchfield, stay away from people, especially small children. Well, I already canceled Thanksgiving dinner at my mother's, we'll just be at home in New York tomorrow, but we were planning to go to Litchfield on Friday. And we're giving a cocktail party with my mother on Saturday, at her house. I don't think you ought to go. Your white count will probably go lower still, and I don't think it's safe. Also, you should cancel whatever you have scheduled early next week, stay out of Roosevelt Hospital, where you might be exposed to sick people, stay away from patients. Okay. You know, we're planning to go to Vail to ski in ten days. Oh, Cesca, I don't think you should do that.

Damn, I really want to go to Vail, but now Anne has me worried. White cells at 900, only 25 percent the kind that fight bacteria. That is very low, I concede to myself. I call the hotel, tell them I have to have some surgery, change the reservation so just Bill has a place to stay. They are fairly gracious about it, may be able to give us a refund if they can fill the space.

Heather and J are home for Thanksgiving, and for the first time ever, we are going to have Thanksgiving dinner at home, just the four of us. We all want it to be a special day, it's kind of Thanksgiving and Christmas all rolled into one, and, though we don't talk about it, we know it might be the last.

We decide to do it in the middle of the day. The housekeeper has done the shopping, but I forgot about the stuffing. Early in the morning I consult my cookbooks, find a recipe for sausage stuffing, and pick up the ingredients in the deli-grocery across the street. I make the stuffing, Jim and J stuff the bird after I admonish them that it's important not to pack the stuffing in too hard, just let it fall in. Then when I see so much stuffing not in the bird, I surreptitiously jam it all in and Jim bursts out laughing when he sees me. It's a very lighthearted moment.

J takes over the basting duties, and Jim and I go for a walk in the park. The weather is sunny and mild, and in all that fresh air I don't think I'll be exposed to sick people. We walk for miles, hand in hand, down around the boat pond, into the Ramble, back across the playing fields, and up toward the reservoir. A lovely walk, we're both refreshed and relaxed when we get home.

Heather has emerged from the long sleep of the college student, and the turkey is nearly done. We decide to use all the best stuff. Heather polishes the silver, flatware, serving dishes, and we set the table. I make the vegetables, and J shows great interest in the gravy. We make it together, I show him all my secrets, and he takes over authoritatively. Okay, Gravymaster.

We open a bottle of champagne, sip it while the four of us crowd into the tiny kitchen, assembling the feast. We are caught up in the fun. We sit down together to eat. The pale November sun floods the table, glinting off the crystal, the gleaming silver, our children's sandy blond hair. We toast the day, raising glasses silently, wordlessly willing that this will not be the last. I am suffused with joy, surrounded by my family, drenched in their love. I am grateful. If this is all that's to be, it is enough.

The meal is fabulous, we all pig out. No one has room for the pecan pie. We decide to take a break before dessert. Heather and J go to the video store and return with a favorite, *Ghostbusters*. We watch together, we've seen this so many times we can anticipate all our favorite lines, and we do, doubling over in laughter time and again.

I get my blood counts checked again Friday morning, because Anne anticipated they would be even lower now. Good news, the white count is up to 1.2, which means I've bottomed out and am on the upswing. I persuade Anne that going to Litchfield will be safe, I'll stay away from little children, and I won't kiss anyone hello at the cocktail party. And if I feel lousy, I won't go. Okay, Cesca, but come right back to New York if you get a fever, or sore throat, or anything.

The weekend is uneventful, I feel fine, see all our friends at the cocktail party, and even if I'm a bit stand-offish, no one notices.

I notice some hot flashes, that's what it must be, a sudden rush of heat and sense of sweltering in a cool room. I guess the ovaries are starting to go. I don't like it, forty-two is too young for menopause, yet this is not entirely unexpected, really, when I think about it, why else do the chemotherapy pamphlets suggest one may become sterile? The irony is overwhelming—a year ago I was trying to figure out the best way to get sterilized. Be careful what you ask for, I think darkly, you may get it, but from an entirely different direction. I wanted to be sterile, not castrated.

The wig situation is not good. I'm not very happy with my new wig, and I've been reading a magazine article about very high-priced professional real-hair wigs. It sounds like something I better check out soon, because I sense my hair is going to thin out rapidly after this last big blast of chemo. I enlist J, tell him I want him to come with me when I go see these people on Monday, because his sandy blond hair color is very close to my original mousy dark blond color, and they'll need samples to match. Okay, Mom, very little enthusiasm, but he agrees to come. J asks me questions about the transplant. I give him the copy of the protocol to read. No more questions.

DECEMBER 1986

On Monday we go to a couple of custom-made-wig places. One is significantly better than the other, and I choose the place run by a warm and sympathetic woman. J tolerates her lavish praise of his beautiful hair, and she takes samples from different parts of his head, explaining that everyone's hair is darker at the back, lighter on top, and that's one of the things that makes her wigs look so natural. She takes about twenty-seven different measurements of my head to make the base, and we schedule two more appointments for fittings and approval of the hair that she will make it from. The finished product won't be ready for at least three weeks, maybe four. Will it stay on? Yes. Can I sleep in it? Sure, many people do. I hope it will be ready in time for me to take to the hospital.

My white blood cell count on Monday is up to 2. I start to reconsider going to Vail—I really want to go. I lobby Anne, tell her I think my counts are coming back fast, and why not go to Vail? She's cautious, says that I really don't have enough polys, the bacterial fighters, to be safe. Well, how many polys do I need? About a thousand, and right now you only have 120. Oh. But if it comes back by the end of the week, I could go, right? Well, let's see how it goes; I don't think they're going to come back that fast.

I fly to Boston early on Tuesday for another bone marrow, and the lung and heart function tests required by the treatment protocol. Ken does bilateral bone marrows, two are always worse than one, but the other tests are not painful. The lung tests involve breathing into tubes in various ways, like the ones we did in physiology class way back in medical school, in addition to blood drawn from an artery rather than a vein to measure how much oxygen I get into my blood.

The heart function test is much more sophisticated than an EKG stress test and gives the kind of information previously available only with cardiac catheterization. It's a boring test for me, actually; all I do is get an injection of a radioactive substance that tags red blood cells, wait twenty minutes, and then lie under a scanner pointed at my heart with EKG leads taped to my chest. Through some incredibly complicated computerized process, the machine figures out how much blood is pumped out of the ventricles with each heartbeat, what they call the ejection fraction. The more efficient heart pumps more of what's in the ventricle. Ken tells me in the afternoon that I must be in terrific shape because the doctor evaluating the test asked him if I was an athlete! My ejection fraction was 76 percent, normal is about 50 percent. I am absurdly pleased by this result; all the exercise I've been doing is accomplishing something after all.

When will you know for sure about the harvest date? We'll know better next week, but I won't be here, Ken says, I have to go to the annual meeting of blood component lab directors, but you can call Jerry Ritz at the end of next week. Okay, I might just be in Vail skiing, but I can call from there. Skiing? There's a meeting there I want to go to, and it'll be our last vacation for a long time, I really want to go, and Anne says if my polys come up by the end of the week I can. We'd be leaving Sunday, that should be plenty of time for them to come back enough. Well, just don't get hurt. Ken is suddenly worried that I might break a leg on the eve of the transplant, he's like a mother hen. I laugh. Don't worry, I'm a very careful skier, the original chicken.

On Wednesday morning I talk with Jim about the trip

to Vail, which we've canceled, can he go if I get the go-ahead later this week? I don't think there will be too much trouble reinstating our reservations. Jim demurs, not because he can't change his plans back, but because he thinks I'm trying to do too much. Just let it be, Cesca, we don't need to go, just stay home and relax. I want to go. Jim flares, You want too much!

I burst into tears. I have given up so much! I've lost my ovaries, I'm losing my hair, I'm losing my work, I have to leave you and the kids and my friends and everything behind and go away, and you want me to give up this week of skiing! You think I want too much, and I've lost everything!? I storm into Heather's room, sit on her bed, and sob in rage. In a few minutes Jim walks in, remorse large on his face. I'm so sorry, I had no idea about your ovaries and all. He sits next to me and hugs me. We'll go if we can, he says.

Later in the day, in the office, George Zambetti comes in and sits down. He must have something on his mind, because he usually doesn't just drop in for idle chitchat. He asks how I'm going to handle my absence from work as far as the practice is concerned. I don't know, George, I've been thinking about it a lot, but so far all I've come up with is a sabbatical. I'll tell my patients I'm going on a sabbatical, but I don't know if other doctors are going to buy that—I'm worried that there may be a lot of rumor-mongering about what's really going on. He reminds me of a letter we got from an internist a few years ago who was retiring for medical reasons, how clear and simple it was, everyone got the message at once, there were clear-cut plans for his patients' follow-up, and though everyone was surprised and talked about it for a day or so, the news passed swiftly without rumors and gossip. I get it at once, how simple. Yes, that would probably be the best way, George, just tell the truth. Thank you for thinking of this, I've really been stuck, but this feels so right. George smiles an embarrassed smile. Just happy to be of help.

I start to write the letter immediately. It's incredibly easy to write the truth, and a relief. I'll hold off on sending it out until I'm actually in the hospital for the transplant, because although I'm ready to tell the truth about what's happening, I'm not ready to face my colleagues' shock, face-to-face. And I think they will be shocked when they get this letter:

Dear Colleague,

I am writing to tell you that I am on a medical leave of absence from my practice until spring. Last spring I learned that I have multiple myeloma. The initial chemotherapy has produced a complete clinical remission. I have decided to undergo autologous bone marrow transplantation to produce a permanent cure. On the advice of my physician, this will require a leave of absence from my practice for about three or four months.

In the meantime, Ruth O'Sullivan, my secretary, will be in the office to triage my patients' problems; acute or urgent problems will be handled by my six partners and I will be in constant communication with Ruth and my six partners about less urgent patient concerns. Bill Hamilton will cover the Tuesday afternoon adult orthopaedic clinic at Roosevelt Hospital. If you have any elective referrals, Drs. Patterson and Hamilton will be able to care for them.

I look forward to resuming active practice and surgery in March or April.

Sincerely yours,
Francesca M. Thompson, M.D.

This letter feels right to me, straightforward and to the point. It suggests a beginning and an end to my leave of absence, and then when I do come back, if I do come back—of course I will come back—I can send another letter out announcing the resumption of my practice. I show my rough draft to my partners, ask them what they think. They all like it except Charlie, who suggests that I don't have to explain anything, it's nobody's business but my own. I tell Charlie I think this way is better, because there will be a lot of talk and unfounded speculation if I just disappear. People will be asking him and the other partners what's going on, and the truth is much easier to deal with than made-up stories.

I walk home from the office on Wednesday and am overwhelmed by fatigue. I think to myself that maybe Jim is right, maybe going to Vail will be too tiring, I couldn't ski if I felt like this. I call Anne when I get home, ask her if something could be wrong with my thyroid or something. I'm so exhausted, maybe the chemo knocked out my thyroid and that's why I'm tired. No, I don't think so, Cesca, I think it's just that your counts are so low, people feel very tired when the counts are low.

I rest all day Thursday. I'm still under orders to stay out of contact with patients, although I cheated a little yesterday in the office. On Friday morning, on my way to the hotel for the foot and ankle course, I stop for another blood count. This will tell if I can go or not, I'll get the results in a couple of hours. During the first break, I go to the phones, get my white count, 2.9, 25 percent polys. That's almost 750. I call Anne, she is surprised it's come up so fast and agrees readily that by Sunday it will be fine. I can go to Vail!

I call the hotel, they are accomodating, Yes, you can have a two-bedroom condo with Dr. Hamilton, but it will be in another building from the original reservation. That's okay. I confirm the plane reservations and reserve a bus from Denver to Vail. I am thrilled that it's all falling together.

I give a brief talk on Saturday, relieved that I still have my hair and don't have to wear the unsatisfactory wig.

Maybe I won't lose my hair after all. I don't feel tired any-more, even staying out late at the faculty dinner.

On Sunday Jim and I catch the morning flight to Den-ver. On the plane I notice that I'm shedding hair all over my coat. I'm shedding like a collie in the spring. Shit, it's happening. I pull tentatively on a small hank of hair, it all comes out in my fingers. Good thing I packed my wigs. The rest of the plane trip I can think of almost nothing but my hair. Is this it?

As soon as we settle into our condo, I unpack and get into the shower to wash my hair. It comes out from the pressure of the shower, sticks to my body in strands, ent-wines in my fingers. Within minutes, all my hair is gone, clogging the drain, and I am bald, almost totally bald, just a few pathetic hairs here and there looking grotesque against my pink, shiny scalp. I look in the steamy mirror, swipe at it with a towel, and cry. I am shocked at what I see—a cancer patient, a dying woman. How can I look so terrible, and feel okay?

Jim takes it well, doesn't act repelled, even tries to get me to laugh. My sense of humor has deserted me. I try on my wigs, it's command decision time, which one should I wear, the reddish one or the mousy one with touches of gray hair? Jim likes the mousy one. I prefer the one with-out the gray, and put it on, trying to brush it into some-thing resembling my style, but it keeps slipping off, this is going to take some practice. I'm in tears again, picture my-self in some public ladies' room, knocking my wig off in front of everyone.

Bill Hamilton shares the condo with us. We enlist him in the wig decision in the morning, which do you think is better? He's very diplomatic, and just showing him my dif-ferent wigs makes me feel better, more down-to-earth and practical, less caught up in my loss. I decide to just wear a tight wool cap with long braids of wool hanging down on either side, the newest style in ski hats. I like it, it feels like hair.

The meetings are scheduled at eight in the morning and four in the afternoon, and they are so good we actually run longer in the mornings. We are a group of friends both at the meetings and on the slopes, where we ski and lunch together, and then we have dinner at various restaurants at night. The week passes swiftly, everyone is having a marvelous time. In my hat with the braids, I guess I'm the only person who doesn't ever take my hat off in the lodge at lunch. My energy level is very high, and I can ski longer and harder than ever before. It's fun sharing the condo with Bill. Jim and I relax with him after skiing, sipping drinks and lazing around before dinner.

The hot flashes get worse and are particularly trying at dinner, where I learn to hang on to my menu so I can use it as a fan. Joan Mann is having similar difficulties, and we laugh together as we take off sweaters in a cool room or fan our menus at dinner. One evening Joan and Roger have a cocktail party at their condo before dinner. Several of Roger's former fellows have come to this meeting, and Jim leans over to me and says, Every single one of Roger's fellows here is bald. We laugh together, sharing the joke.

On Thursday I call Jerry Ritz from the pay phone at the mountaintop lodge at lunchtime. I ask him about the harvest, is it a go? He's very vague, seems not to know that it's been set up, says it has to be discussed with the whole transplant group at their weekly conference, suggests I call Ken on Monday when he's back. Uh-oh, a fly in the ointment. I feel vaguely disquieted. Are they jerking me around? I'm getting all set to go for this transplant soon, are they going to be ready in Boston?

After dinner Friday night I say good-bye to Roger and Joan, they are leaving early in the morning and I won't see them then. It's poignant. We all know I won't see them again for a long time, if ever. Big hugs. I am so choked up I can't speak. Roger, my mentor, my friend, hugs me, says, Hang in there, old girl, be tough. I want to thank him for all he has done for me but I can't get any words out at all.

Back in New York on Monday, I call Ken to find out what's happening. I can't get any definite answer, the transplant beds are full, no point in doing the harvest this week, probably better in a week or so. I'm in an indefinite holding pattern. It's hard to know what to schedule in the office. Might as well schedule things, then cancel later if it works out that way. Not that I really think we can get the harvest organized during Christmas week, no, it'll probably be after Christmas, even after New Year's.

I get Ruth to type up the Dear Colleague letter. I start going through my phone numbers, figuring who should get the letter, the envelopes can be typed in advance. I have decided to tell the women in the office this week. The letter is a convenient prop. I call them in to talk to me, singly or in pairs, two friends together. I give them the letter to read, explaining that I want them to know about this, but to keep it an office secret for now. I answer all their questions, accept their best wishes, and when they ask me what they can do for me, I ask them to watch out for my patients while I'm away, but on the whole, as far as patients are concerned, I'll be on a sabbatical till spring. By Wednesday I've talked to everyone, and I feel better to have it done with; their support has been unreserved. I also let my partners know they can tell their wives, but I don't want this to get out generally till I leave.

On Thursday Ken calls me again, they had a full conference on my case with the transplant group, and everyone is very enthusiastic about my being the first patient on the new myeloma protocol. . . . He hesitates. Only— Only what? I interrupt. Everyone thinks it would be better if you have another consolidation course of Cytoxan, and this time, also high-dose dexamethasone. Oh, no, I think, not again! Why? I ask. I thought the protocol was that after you're in remission, you get one consolidation course, and then the transplant. Yes, Ken agrees, but everyone, Lee Nadler, particularly, and he's the one who's had the most experience with the B-cell lymphoma patients, feels that the patients who had two courses of consolidation therapy did better than the ones who had just one, but we don't have big enough numbers to prove it statistically.

And then what? I say. Are you going to call me and say everyone thinks you're doing really great, and you'll do even better if you have a third round of consolidation therapy? Listen, the reason I want this transplant is that we know repeated cycles of chemo don't cure it and can eventually cause other cancers. What is the end point?

No, no, Ken assures me. Just this one more round, there won't be any more. Where would we do it? You can come up here, or do it in New York. I want to talk to Anne, I'll call you back. Ken says he'll have Lee Nadler call me too.

I call Anne, tell her what they have just suggested. What do you think, Anne? Cesca, they're the ones to call the shots in this, as far as I'm concerned, if they say jump, we say, How high? I groan inwardly, remembering the days of nausea, the incapacitation of the last consolidation round. They want me to do it in one fell swoop in the hospital, and with a shitload of dexamethasone, too; can you do that at New York Hospital? Well, that's not the way we usually do it, but I can talk to them and follow their protocol. But can you get me a bed right away at New York Hospital? That might be more of a problem, but I think I can get one on Saturday. Okay, I'll talk to Ken again and get back to you.

I look at the calendar and start calculating. This sets the whole transplant back by five weeks. That would be, let's see, about January 22 before I'd be ready for the harvest, to give my marrow time to come back fully. I suddenly brighten, that means I could go to the Foot Society meeting and the Academy meeting for my induction in San Francisco if we just wait another week to do the harvest. The meetings are from Wednesday the twenty-first through the weekend.

Lee Nadler calls. He's the one who invented the first of

the three antibodies that's going to be used to clean up my marrow. I haven't met him yet, but I know Ken has had him call me because Lee is supposed to be the tough guy, the one to persuade me to do what they want. I've already decided to do it anyway—I have no choice, as Anne pointed out—but I let him give his pitch. I listen, thinking to myself that I better go along with what they recommend, I wouldn't want to go through the whole transplant and have it not work, and have them able to say that I should have had the second consolidation round. Ditto the dexamethasone, which scares me, such a huge dose. Hey, I say to Lee, I don't want to get aseptic necrosis of my hips. Look, he says, if you're alive in four or five years, and then you get aseptic necrosis of your hips, at least you'll be alive, and we'll all be happy about that. But it's such a huge dose. Yeah, you'll probably be in orbit someplace.

I call Ken back, discuss the alternatives of New York versus Boston. He can easily get me a bed, I can come up on Saturday, go home Monday morning. Okay, that sounds the simplest. I'd rather be in the hospital where the nurses are used to the treatment plan, don't feel they're winging something new on the weekend.

We arrive in Boston via the shuttle by early afternoon. The hospital seems deserted, but the skeleton crew get me checked in, send me around to the labs for the routine EKG, chest X ray, and blood tests. Ken had already told me he wouldn't be there till late afternoon or early evening, but he's left all the admission orders, and the nurses tell me everything is all set for the chemo. But actually they don't start it till nighttime, because they plan to use high doses of intravenous Nembutal, a strong barbiturate, so I can sleep through the worst of it. I give them my own supply of Marinol, explain that I've had better nausea control with the marijuana, what they call THC, than anything else.

Ken comes by in the late afternoon and we go over the whole treatment regimen. I'll get everything by intravenous. The nearly five grams of Cytoxan, what I had in divided doses over four days on the last round, will be given over one hour. The dexamethasone will be IV as well, I guess so they can be sure of the dose, no good if I throw it up. Because the initial breakdown products of the Cytoxan in such a high dose are so damaging to the bladder, I will have constant bladder irrigation by means of a catheter, with an inflow tube as well as an outflow tube. Yuck. Also useful because the intravenous fluids will be at such a high level that if I didn't have the catheter I'd be getting up to pee all night, and they want me to be zonked out.

Jim and I watch TV. The room is pleasant and modern, very self-contained, but the mattress is hard, and the pillow is noisy, wrapped in stiff waterproof plastic. I make a mental note to bring my own pillows next time. After supper, Jim goes home with his sister Betsy, who comes by to visit.

Around nine P.M. the nurses get me to change into a hospital gown and insert the catheter, and then the IV. They start the zonking medication along with a liter of plain fluid. I nod out, spend a restless night twisting and turning, throwing up, and complaining about everything, especially the catheter, which, although it is working well, makes me feel an urgent need to pee all the time. The nurses escalate the doses of Nembutal, Trilafon, Ativan, which I seem to be soaking up without much effect.

By morning, when Jim arrives, I'm a wreck. I've gotten some pajama bottoms, but the top keeps twisting around, my wig won't stay on and I've given it up. Breakfast holds no appeal, so Jim eats my meal, which is useful because the cafeteria is closed on weekends. The day spins by. I am roused to consciousness to throw up and take these opportunities to complain to the nurse that her best stuff isn't working well. We've already added the THC, and it isn't working too well either. I have a vague awareness of Ken and my cousin Karen and Cox coming by for a visit; I wish they would just go away and leave me alone, which I guess they do.

I get rid of the damn catheter and sleep through the night heavily drugged. It's a good rest, I wake up Monday morning totally alert and ready to roll. We want to get out as soon as possible so Jim can get to work. I dress and pack right away. Ken is surprised to see me recovered so fast but has no objection to my leaving immediately. He gives me a prescription for two more doses of 80 milligrams of dexamethasone, and we joke about how high I'll be flying on this. I've figured out that this is equivalent to over 500 milligrams of prednisone, and we think of 100 milligrams of prednisone as being a fairly high dose. The highest I've had so far is 60 milligrams, so this is eight times that. Wow! No wonder I feel so good today, steroids are one of the real feel-good drugs. I hope the crash won't be too hard when I come off it.

I even go to the office Monday afternoon, catch up on phone calls, paperwork, and arrange to see a few patients the following day. Heather and J are home on vacation. We all do a little shopping, but by common consent this is not supposed to be a big gift-giving Christmas, because I'm supposed to stay out of the stores and crowds. Jim and I have never exchanged surprise presents anyway, we prefer to get something together, and this agreement has saved a lot of disappointment about not being able to read each other's minds over the years.

My big present is my new wig, and it's ready on Christmas Eve. It's very nice in color, but the style is more soignée than my hair usually is. It will take some getting used to. But it looks very real, subtle variations in color, real hair texture, no gray. I guess I like it. At least it's better than the synthetic wig I've been wearing.

We plan a quiet long weekend from Wednesday to Sunday in Litchfield. Betsy comes down from Boston to join us. We put out the presents Wednesday night; there seem to be a large number for me. On Thursday morning I find out why. Jim gives me a portable compact disc player to take to the hospital, and a large starter selection of my favorite classical pieces. I am very touched. Jim broke our rule, but I am pleased, feel cosseted by his thoughtfulness. My other favorite present from Jim is a small Japanese fan, a delightful way to cope with the hot flashes, which are getting worse and worse.

On Friday I start taking an antibiotic as prophylaxis, prevention, against bacterial infection during the anticipated nadir of my counts. This is somewhat controversial: some oncologists prefer to wait until a fever signals that an infection has become established and to check the blood counts with frequent blood tests; that was how Anne and I did it last time. Ken, however, recommended this five-day course of antibiotics to keep me on the safe side over the holiday weekend, when getting to a place for blood tests would be difficult. Anne is willing to go along with it but is careful to let me know where to find her all weekend, and she makes me promise to come to New York immediately if I develop a fever.

I feel fine all weekend and even chance an appearance at a large cocktail party, where several friends, mostly women, comment on my new hairstyle with great enthusiasm. One woman, a friend from childhood, exclaims that if she found a hairdresser like mine she'd hang on to him forever. I smile obliquely, say, I think I'll do just that, enjoying my private joke.

It's easier to worry about my hair than think about my impending separation from the real world. Jim has been bugging me about how we're going to handle this with our friends. When he asks what he's supposed to say when people call me at home when I'm in the hospital, I avoid the issue. Just say I can't come to the phone right now, get their number, and then call me, and I'll call them back. He gives me a quizzical look. I know what he means, it's nutty. Look, Jim says, you're putting me in a very awkward situation, people are going to think we're separated or something. Well, I say evasively, we will be separated. Jim gives me another one of those looks, his patience is wearing thin.

I think about it. He's right. We're going to have to come clean about this. Actually, there's no way I can send that letter out to my colleagues and not have word of my illness get out to our friends in Litchfield. A few of the doctors on my list go to Litchfield on weekends, many more have patients from Litchfield. Bad news travels fast, and this will get out. But I don't want it to get out until I'm already beyond the point of no return in the hospital. There are two couples I want to tell in person, they've been our closest friends in Litchfield for many years. I resolve to tell both this weekend and I do, in person, dropping in unexpectedly after lunch on Saturday. After absorbing the initial shock, they are full of offers of help to Jim and the children, focusing their concern on all of us.

When I get home, Jim asks how it went. Fine, I say. I can sense that Jim is relieved that I have gotten over this hurdle, and that he has friends now he can share this trouble with. I realize I have left him isolated from outside comfort. Hardly anyone knows what he's going through, except the family and a couple of friends at his office he has chosen to confide in. I really have been pretty selfish in my single-minded pursuit of secrecy, my desire to keep the world from knowing I am vulnerable, so vulnerable I might die. I can see the change in Jim at a cocktail party that night where both couples spend some time privately with Jim. He is more relaxed and expansive than he has been lately.

On Monday morning in Litchfield, I close on a mortgage of our house, a move I have orchestrated to pay off my education debts drawn against Jim's pension fund and transfer them to my estate, some more getting my affairs in order, just in case. I don't want Jim left with my debts against his name when my life insurance will cover a mortgage.

On Monday my white count is a whopping 1000. I must have hit bottom sometime over the weekend and am now on the rise. I'm supposed to stay away from patients, but I have a few postoperative patients I really need to see, so I do anyway. I think I'm safe.

I've been wearing my wig constantly, even sleeping in it, trying to make it be my real hair. It looks ratty now, and I go see the wig woman to complain. You said I could treat this like my own hair, and look at it, it's terrible! She looks at me with wide eyes. But you have to set it. Set it? I've never set my hair, how do you do that? Patiently, she demonstrates. See, you put on the chinstrap, small alligator clamps on either side by the ears so it won't fall off, spritz it with some water with a little conditioner in it, then twist a hank into a small circle and clip it in place. It'll dry in a little while, then take the clips out and brush it lightly. See? I see. Back to the fifties, no more casual disregard of hair, towel drying after showers.

My new wig does not go unnoticed at the hospital. One morning in the surgeons' lounge a young plastic surgeon looks over at me as I'm reading the paper and chatting with Bill and Fiske. Hey, Cesca, she exclaims loudly enough for the whole room to hear, your hair looks different, it's really nice, what did you do? Without a second's hesitation I tell her, We finally got the color right, letting a note of exasperation and impatience at the imperfections of hairdressers slip into my voice.

I start making plans for my last month of freedom. After spending so many months wanting desperately to get on with this, I feel secretly relieved to have it postponed, and it's not my fault, I didn't chicken out, they insisted on the second consolidation chemotherapy, my reprieve.

I receive a letter from the guy who is going to be president of the Foot and Ankle Society this year, telling me that he's appointed me to the chairmanship of an important committee. I feel flattered, and wonder only briefly if I should accept. Of course I should, I can do the paperwork in the hospital, no sweat. The letter goes on to detail the time and place of the meeting of the board of directors, which I should attend at the conference in San Francisco.

Uh-oh, it's the same time as the induction ceremony at the academy meeting, the one Charlie has been insisting we attend together. Looks like I'll have to decide between them. Well, I'll decide later.

I confirm with Ken that the harvest will be on January 29, a Thursday, and we'll hope a bed will be available in the transplant unit on Saturday, which is the day of the week they like to start the transplant regimen, so that the radiation therapy can be given on weekdays instead of on the weekend. Also, Ken says, you need to come up again before then because we need to store your marrow in your own plasma, and to do that we need to draw the blood ahead of time so we can spin it down, extract the plasma, and have it ready when we treat your marrow the day of the harvest. And we have to test your blood for a lot of antibodies. We decide on January 26, the day after I get back from San Francisco.

I tell Ken I want to rent a place locally for Jim to stay. Although he could stay at his sister's, her place is a long drive from the hospital, and it would be more convenient for him to have a place nearby. Any ideas? Ken suggests I call him back about that after the holidays. He thinks the social worker can help with that, but better wait for now, there will be plenty of time to arrange that in the early part of January.

⋮

JANUARY 1987

⋮

These hot flashes are getting ridiculous, intolerable. I talk to Anne about it, ask her if there would be any reason not to take estrogen. No, no reason at all, in fact, why suffer? Within a few days of starting estrogen replacement, the hot flashes disappear, and my hand-held fan is relegated to the back of the closet, no longer needed.

I resume my exercise, having suspended it while my counts were down. I start slowly, just two kilometers at first on the cross-country machine, and walking to the office. It's hard to get into it again, but I force myself, want to maintain that fantastic aerobic capacity I had last month on the ventricular scan. If I don't exercise this month, I could lose a lot of the conditioning I had. After a few days of ski-machining, I return to the one-on-one exercise sessions. It wipes me out. I feel like fainting, have to lie down on the mat for awhile till my heart rate recovers. My trainer is concerned, but I dismiss it, saying only that I've sort of been down with the flu lately, and I guess I'm weaker than I thought. I'll slow down. I quit the session early, but schedule one for later in the week.

My work schedule is very light, little or no surgery, and fewer patients than usual. I'm getting concerned about it, but what do I expect? For the last six weeks I've been on-again, off-again, totally unable to count on being there, often changing appointments with patients at the last minute to accommodate a trip to Boston or threatened illness because of chemotherapy. It's just no way to run a practice. Furthermore, I've been careful to explain to patients who want surgery that I'll be leaving soon on a sabbatical, and they can wait till I come back, have me do the surgery, and see one of my partners for the follow-up visits, or they can have one of my partners take care of them, which is the course I recommend to those who don't want to wait till I get back.

Now that my white count is back to normal, I have to get my teeth checked. Ken has emphasized the importance of making sure that I have no dental problems, incipient abscesses, or residual plaque that could go haywire, cause a life-threatening infection during the time of no white cells. After a couple of sessions with my dentist, I get the all clear; yes, I'll need some periodontal work in the future, but my teeth shouldn't do me in during the transplant.

With Ken's help, I get in touch with the social worker at Dana-Farber, who refers me to a nearby apartment-hotel complex just a few minutes' walk from the hospital. They have a two-bedroom furnished apartment we can rent by the month, yes, we could move in on January 28, the day before the scheduled harvest. I send them a check for the first month's rent, sight unseen. Good, now we have a home base in Boston.

I ask Ken about exercising while I'm in the hospital, is it feasible to use a cross-country ski machine instead of the stationary bike you told me about? Oh, sure, I think that would be okay. Then I'll order one and have it sent to you; I'll use it while I'm in the hospital, and then I'll donate it to the hospital for other patients to use. Okay, great.

I start to collect things I want to take to the hospital. Lots of books, professional reading I haven't gotten around to, novels, data to write clinical papers. I'll be able to get a lot done. Tapes and compact discs. Heather's portable radio. A VCR tape of the Mets stunning season, Ken has told me they have a VCR machine available to patients. Clothes to exercise in, shorts and sweats. My hospital scrub suits, I've decided they would be the most comfortable thing to wear, I learned in my last admission that the hospital gowns are a disaster, the snaps don't work, and as I toss and turn, I get choked around the neck by them as they ride up. A bathrobe, sandals, running shoes. Writing paper, I've ordered a supply. And pillows, I've got to take up a couple of good pillows.

I think about what the time in the hospital will be like. Ken has said again and again that the hard part will be coping with the boredom and confinement after the expected two weeks of unpleasant side effects of radiochemotherapy. I hope I've thought of enough things to keep me occupied constructively. I'll have to make a schedule for myself, get through each day that way, so much time for exercise, so much time for heavy-duty reading, so much time for light reading, letter writing. Think of all I can get done with a little organization!

I go over my will with Pete Goodwin, Charlie's father, again, and by now I've told him of my plans for the hospital. There are some technicalities with different trust arrangements he'd like to fine-tune, he'll get another will prepared to sign before I go. Meanwhile, I prepare a number of powers of attorney for Jim.

My godson's wedding is Saturday evening, the reception a dinner dance. Jim and I have been very close to the groom's father for over twenty years, in fact, he is J's godfather. Despite the happy occasion, there is an undercurrent of sadness because our friend's marriage is breaking up, his separation will occur soon. In quiet conversations with other longtime friends, we talk about our distress that his marriage has gone awry in the year of his fiftieth birthday, which we know is a big deal for him, and come up with a plan to throw him a fiftieth birthday party ourselves, a surprise party. I think to myself that for sure I'll be recovered by mid-May, and helping to plan a nice party for our friend will give me something to do. By the end of the evening we have five couples altogether who will host this event. I get the orchestra leader's card because we'd like to do a dinner dance, and these guys are good.

My anxiety level is rising steadily, I start smoking an occasional cigarette. By the time I fly to San Francisco for the meetings, I buy a pack, smoke in my room. What the hell? I like it, and I'll stop, of course, when I go in the hospital, just as I'll give up alcohol, chocolate, fresh fruit, salads, probably any kind of food I like because of the special bacteria-free diet. Might as well enjoy myself now.

I think about the transplant when I'm alone. I realize that out here in San Francisco it seems so remote, so unreal. It's hard for me to believe it's really going to happen, that in just over a week's time, I'll leave New York and my real life behind. The lack of reality insulates me from fear, but every now and then it breaks through, and I can admit it. I'm scared, scared of dying up there on the transplant unit in Boston. No, I quickly tell myself, you're not going to die up there.

The busyness of the Foot Society meeting and related social events keeps my mind off macabre thinking. I concentrate on the future beyond the transplant, and when I have to decide whether to go to the induction ceremony and sit with my friends from the studying-for-the-boards period while we listen to a speech welcoming us into the American Academy of Orthopaedic Surgeons, or go to the Foot Society board of directors meeting to learn what my committee chairmanship should be about, I opt for the latter. It is a statement to myself: I intend to be around to do this job in the future; look forward, not back, that's what's important to me now. Later, when I see my partner Charlie Goodwin, he says, Where the hell were you, I looked all over for you, we all missed you and I thought something was wrong! Gee, I'm sorry, Charlie, I had to be at this Foot Society meeting at the same time, and I didn't know how to get word to you. It's a lame excuse, and I feel guilty for letting him down.

I leave San Francisco on Saturday, changing my plane reservations from Sunday when I realize I would miss the Giants in the Super Bowl if I fly then. I want to watch the game with Jim. This could be the year of wins: the Mets, maybe the Giants, how about me, too? I don't want to admit to superstitious thinking, but these things get hooked up in my mind. Magic, I could use some magic. Yes, of course the Giants win the Super Bowl; yes, of course I'll do great up there in Boston.

I have to go to Boston Monday to give them blood so they can prepare the plasma to store my marrow in after they treat it with the antibodies. The weather report Sunday night is for bad weather the next day, so I get up early, rush out to the airport in heavy snow to grab the first shuttle out, I've got to get there before they close the airport. In my rush to lock the car, I drop my car keys in the snow. Great! Now I have to taxi home this afternoon, get the extra keys at home, taxi back to the car. Well, forget it for now, just get on the plane.

Boston is hit hard by the snowstorm by the time I get there. No cabs. I grab the airport bus, hoping to find someplace where there are more cabs, learn from the other passengers that the subway would be a good way to get there. They tell me which line I want, and I follow them. At the transfer station, a large crowd develops, none of the trains I want is coming along. After a half-hour wait, the dispatcher announces that a breakdown has blocked that line for the foreseeable future. Oh, no!

I head above ground, surface in a blizzard in the middle of Boston. The man at the newsstand points to a taxi stand at a nearby hotel, maybe I can find one there. I hail a cab pulling out of the stand, he has a passenger, but they're allowed to double up in snow emergencies. We pick up another fare heading in the direction of Brookline and drop off first one, then the other. The driver seems resigned to a bad day in the snow. I make a deal with him to wait for me at Dana-Farber while I get my blood drawn, shouldn't take long at all, and then he can take me back to the airport.

I arrive at the hospital and check in at the clinic. And wait. And wait. I start hassling the women at the desk, Look, I've got a cab waiting for me, I've got to get out before they shut the airport, I'm just here for a blood test, can't someone else do it if you can't find Felice, the transplant nurse? No response. I go to a phone and page Ken. He is surprised to hear my voice, where are you? I'm right here in the clinic, have been for half an hour, and nobody knows what's happening, Felice isn't here, and drawing my blood isn't in their job description! Plus I have a cab waiting outside to take me back to the airport, I hope he doesn't just disappear. Ken says he'll be right down.

Ken is amazed I am there. Half the hospital staff can't make it in to work, and I've slogged my way in through a big blizzard from New York. As Ken gets me settled in the blood-drawing area, Felice arrives. She takes over drawing huge amounts of blood in large syringes—How much are you taking, anyway? About 500 cc. Wow, I think, that's a lot.

Ken says they want to get another bone marrow today, it's part of the protocol. Wait a second, you said the one in December would be the last. I know I did, but to be complete we're supposed to have one before the harvest. I dig in, obdurate and determined not to have another painful bone marrow for what seems to me to be no good reason at all. I am pissed off and not about to yield. I confront Ken. Do you mean to tell me that given the fact that my bone marrow was totally normal after the consolidation therapy in November, you think that after another huge round of chemo up here in December, somehow the tumor has grown back in the space of a few weeks, do you really think that? No, he admits. I point out that I know the protocol wants bone marrow biopsies taken just before treating the marrow, but those can be obtained on Thursday, painlessly for me, while they're doing the harvest. And further, just on the off chance that the tumor load is too great to do the transplant, they will have the results of Thursday's biopsies before starting the chemo on Sunday. True, Ken admits.

Felice, who has been taking this all in, adds her point of view, saying the cost of harvesting and treating my marrow will be about ten thousand dollars and will be totally wasted if the marrow shows I'm not ready for the transplant. Felice seems hostile to me, clearly regarding me as a spoiled brat who won't cooperate. I've had it with bone marrows, I say, each one hurts more than the last, and this is totally unreasonable. Look, I point out, just a couple of weeks ago the IgG level was down to 850, that's even less than it was in December, so how could the tumor have come back? I ignore Felice, who is still disapproving, and turn to Ken. I don't want another marrow today, but I will consent to one if you tell me honestly that if I don't do it, you'll cancel the transplant. No, he wouldn't do that.

I rush off to find my cab. Ken calls out to me to be careful, please. I turn and see the worry on his face and realize that he doesn't want to lose me, his prize bone marrow candidate, the first one to get the antibody he invented, in a plane crash. We need each other.

On the way to the airport the radio says the airport is closed, but I decide to wait there anyway. Arriving at the shuttle entrance, I ask them how soon the shuttle will run again. We haven't closed. I hop on. We taxi out, spend an hour on the runway, come back, change to the next shuttle, and finally take off. It's been a frustrating day, getting there in a snowstorm, fighting over the bone marrow, and now my keyless car. I crouch down in the snowdrift next to my car, sift through the snow till my gloves are soaked, and finally find the keys next to the rear tire. Whew, at least one nice thing happened today. I make it to my office by two for office hours.

On Tuesday afternoon, Charlie and I talk about my surgery this week. I tell him Chip Moore is the surgeon who'll put in the Hickman catheters. Chip Moore? I went to school with him, we were good friends at Harvard! Charlie calls him right away, chats with him, tells him his partner is coming up for a transplant. I leave while they're still talking, and Charlie tells me later he asked Chip what he thought about the transplant, and Chip said it was definitely the way to go in my case, there were no other options. That's what I'd been telling Charlie all along, but I suspect he had had his reservations. I guess the other partners do, too, although no one has spoken against it, they've listened, and offered whatever support they can.

We go to the ballet Tuesday night, have drinks with Bill Hamilton and Charlie Goodwin beforehand. There have been a lot of good-byes at the office, casual and off-hand, see you in a couple of months. I suspect I may be back next week—if anything can go wrong, it will. Maybe the bed won't be available after all. Maybe they won't get enough marrow for two transplants and will have to do another harvest, Ken has mentioned this as an infrequent, but possible, occurrence. I've been put off so many times, have been on the brink of this transplant so often, that I actually have patients scheduled in the office next week, and an operation on Tuesday. The patient, who really wants me to do this operation before I go on sabbatical and understands that I won't know till a day or so beforehand whether I'll be there to do the surgery, amazingly is willing to hang out with the uncertainty.

On Wednesday morning I go down to my lawyer's office and sign my new will, nothing like waiting till the last moment, but I really didn't have time till now. I meet Jim at home, we're all packed and plan to take the late morning shuttle. Jim goes to the bookstore to stock up. He consumes books and probably will need a bunch to cope with hours of waiting.

The weather is clear and cold for the flight up to Boston. We're traveling with a huge amount of gear. The doorman wishes us a nice vacation as we load it all into a radio cab. In the shuttle lounge, we run into Jim's boss's boss. He asks where we're going on vacation, obviously thinking it's strange to leave on a Wednesday. Jim looks at me with a questioning look, and I bite the bullet. Actually, I say, we're taking me to Boston for treatment of a cancer I have, I'm getting a bone marrow transplant. Jaw drops, but he recovers quickly, wishes me all the best, then he and Jim talk business till his shuttle to Washington is called. There, it's not so hard to say it, after all. But I can sense he thinks I'm a goner.

In Boston we taxi from the airport to the apartment I rented sight unseen. We pull up to an old Tudor-style apartment building that dates back to the early part of the century. The common rooms downstairs are Gothic monsters, huge rooms with oriental rugs, carved dark wood paneling, a long traverse to the antiquated elevator.

Our apartment is a delightful surprise, sun pouring in through bay windows in the living room. The furniture is modern, overstuffed, blond wood, right out of *Metropolitan Home.* The bedrooms are small but adequate, and the dining room is sizable, a relic of the past, situated next to the kitchen, which boasts a freestanding refrigerator, a gas stove, and a dish rack instead of a dishwasher. This will do very nicely, I'm sure, and it will be pleasant to convalesce in a living room flooded with sun in the afternoon.

We load my overnight bag on the schlepper and walk over to Dana-Farber. I meet Felice there. She seems to have gotten over her disapproval of two days ago, gives me paperwork to take to the hospital next door, Brigham and Women's, where the surgery will take place. In addition to the usual admission tests, I have to have some special chest X rays so they can make lead shields to damp down the amount of radiation my lungs get during the total body irradiation.

I get to my room, a pleasant private one, with little fuss. The anesthesiologist comes by to discuss the anesthesia consent. A somber, dour man who never smiles, he and I discuss whether I should get steroids or not. Given the amount I had some weeks ago, it's sort of plus-minus whether I would have adrenal suppression and therefore need a boost of steroids to help me cope with the stress of surgery. We decide to use steroids. I sign the consent.

The radiation team comes by to explain the total body irradiation I'll get next week and get me to sign the consent. I glance over it swiftly, look up at them, and say, You want me to know this could kill me. Yes. And I can get cataracts. Yes. Tell me, this pulmonary problem, how long am I at risk? Just the first four to six weeks. What makes it happen? We don't know, it's not predictable, but we try to reduce the danger by using the lung shields you were measured for today. Okay. I sign.

Chip Moore, my surgeon and Charlie's friend and college classmate, comes by to discuss the surgery he will be doing tomorrow, placing the two Hickman catheters, one on each side of my chest. I ask him where the incisions will be, and how big? Less than an inch, about three inches down from the top of the shoulder, in line with the bra strap. It won't be too noticeable. I tell him I don't want the exit on the front of my chest, because I scar very badly, and I don't want to have to give up V-neck styles. I insist on this, and I realize to myself that he must think I'm nuts to worry about how I'm going to look in clothes, as if I had a whole life ahead of me. Can you tunnel down to my abdomen? I don't wear two-piece bathing suits. Chip gauges the distance. No, our tunneler isn't that long. But the distance to just below my armpit is about right. And the exit scars will be hidden in my bra line. I sign the consent for the axillary placement of bilateral Hickman catheters.

Cox's friend, the clinician who spoke with me at length on my first visit, when I came to check out the transplant, comes by with the consent for the harvest tomorrow, explains that he is the attending in charge in January, that's why he's getting this consent, but Ken will be over later to see me. He and Ken will be doing the harvest tomorrow. I read the consent, look up when I get to the blood transfusion part. I'd rather not have a transfusion, can't you just hold off till you spin down my marrow and give me back my own red cells? Well, we won't give you one unless you need it. Okay, so let's talk about it then. No, we have to have special treated thawed cells ready, and that takes some time, so we like to have them ready in the operating room. This blood is too costly and special to just throw out after it's been thawed.

I'm getting pissed off at this runaround. What you're saying is that you don't know if you need to use blood or not, but once you thaw it, you use it, so everyone gets that unit of blood whether they need it or not, right? He is uncomfortable, we're getting off to a bad start, I'm boxing him in. Look, I say, I want real answers to my questions, not some bullshit about how you'll give me blood if I need it when you know you're going to give a unit in the recovery room because it's thawed, and everyone gets a transfusion. I sign the consent, why should I fight over one measly transfusion of a stranger's blood when I'll be getting countless units of red cells and platelets later? But the no-bullshit principle is important to me. I don't want to be jerked around with there-there-dear, nonsense answers.

Ken comes by in the late evening. He will be the attending during February, and we go over the consent for the transplant. This is old hat to me, I've read it numerous times in my copy of the protocol, and sign it readily. Even so, Ken lingers to discuss the possible side effects of the very high doses of intravenous Alkeran I'll be getting. They have not used this before, but he's been checking into the morbidity described by other researchers, and it looks like prolonged, profuse diarrhea is a common result, almost like cholera, vast fluid losses with diarrhea. This sounds unpleasant to me, but not scary. I say, You'll be able to keep up with it with IV fluid replacement, I've had experience in managing sick patients with huge fluid losses, it's no big deal, just push the fluids hard, keep track of the electrolytes. Or, Ken says, you might lose the mucosal layer of your whole GI tract. That might cause a lot of bleeding, I volunteer. Yes. That's what the transfusions are for, but it's a little more worrisome to me. Ken has gotten his message across; they really don't know what this combination of Alkeran and radiation is going to do to me. Behind his words, I sense his anxiety that this may be rough on me, almost a guilty feeling that he will be responsible if something bad happens, something he can't predict or control. I wonder if I should reassure him that it's okay, I won't blame him if things don't go well, but I realize I don't know what's going to happen either.

Jim leaves soon after Ken does, after checking that I should be back in my room in late morning. He is cheerful and positive, not wrung out with anxiety, at least not obviously so, and I am relieved he's taking this in stride, a rock, the one I can lean on.

The nurses wake me for a shot in the early morning dark, and I am very relaxed on my way to the operating room. The nurses let me wear my wig, understand that I don't want to be wheeled down the corridors with my bald head showing. Whatever they give me wipes out consciousness till I wake up in the recovery room, very alert and feeling well. My hips are bound up in thick dressings, as are my shoulders, but there is no pain. I prop myself up. How long do I have to stay here? The nurses are cheerful, A while longer. Do you have anything to read? They find me a newspaper, which I can read without my contact lenses if I hold it close to my nose. I observe the comings and goings of patients and surgeons, it's like all the recovery rooms I've been in before. Finally, I get pushed back to my room.

Jim is all smiles. I hear you've been down there reading and complaining. I wasn't complaining, exactly, I just wanted to leave, it's boring down there, nothing to do. I'm starved, where's lunch? Just then, the tray arrives. Jell-O and broth. No, really, I want real food. The nurse comes in and we negotiate something more substantial.

I spend a fair amount of time on the phone, calling various family members. They are surprised I sound so normal, I guess I am, too, but I feel fine, wide awake and alert, energized really. Jim takes me for a walk, there's a little discomfort, much less than I anticipated. When I climb back into bed, I realize I can't lift my left thigh, I have to lift it up with my hand. Great, somebody bagged the tendon of my rectus femoris muscle on the front of the thigh that attaches to the pointy hip bone in front and plays a large role in raising the leg from the hip. Well, I guess it will heal eventually.

In the late afternoon a large bag of blood arrives from the blood bank; it's my own red cells that have been spun down from the marrow they removed and now will be given back to me. Ken must still be working on treating my marrow, he said it would take all day. I hope they got enough.

By the time Ken arrives it's close to nine at night, and I have already figured out he's late because he doesn't want to tell me there wasn't enough marrow. It went very well, Ken says, we took a huge amount, 1800 cc, that's close to two liters, and it looked like good stuff, with many cells. And? By the time we separated out the cells to treat, there were plenty of cells for one transplant, but not for two. Ken shrugs apologetically. I am not surprised. I figured this would happen. Back on hold. I am so tired of getting all psyched up for this and then getting put off. At least I anticipated this, have some work to do in the office next week.

So when do we do this again? Next week, on Thursday. Déjà vu all over again, as Yogi Berra is wont to say. And I can leave the hospital tomorrow? Yes, I'll see you right after breakfast, and if everything looks good you can go then. What about the bed on the transplant unit, will you hold it for me, or do I have to wait for weeks more? No, we'll have the bed for you.

I call the children, tell them to cancel their plans to come to Boston this weekend, hold off till next week. This is such a bummer, I wanted to get this over with, but in the very far corner of my mind is a small shard of relief: another week of freedom!

We are ready to leave when Ken comes by in the morning. I am moving with little difficulty and have not needed any pain medicine. Ken urges me to get a prescription filled, just in case. I ask Ken if I need to give more blood to spin down plasma to store the marrow in again. Yes, of course, thanks for reminding me, I'll call Felice and you can meet her over at the clinic before you go home.

As Felice draws 500 cc of blood again I think about how absurd this is. In the last five days we've been pouring my blood in and out of me, I'm just a middleman, I think. Jim takes my pillows upstairs to the transplant floor, they have to be sterilized before I can use them, they can get that done this week and they'll be ready for me when I check in next week.

When Jim gets back, Felice fixes me with an authoritarian look and says she is now going to pretend that I am not a doctor, and therefore don't know anything about this, and instructs us in the care of my Hickman catheters, a complex job with sterile gloves, swabs of Betadine and alcohol, and a thin plastic four-by-four-inch occlusive dressing over the spot under each armpit where the thin white Silastic tube exits. Felice has never seen the catheters placed here before, and it does make the dressings more difficult than the usual center-chest placement.

The "lines" themselves, as the catheters are called, have to be flushed daily with small amounts of saline and heparin, so they don't clot off. Jim learns how to do this also, and I pay attention to make sure it's done just as I have always done it. When Felice is satisfied that Jim has learned this ritual, she tells us to pick up our week's supply of catheter equipment in the Dana-Farber pharmacy.

We walk slowly back to Longwood Towers, our apartment-hotel, and when I ascend the steps, I can only climb one step at a time, leading with my right foot, dragging my left. By the time we get there I'm tired, and we decide to rest here overnight and go back to New York in the morning. I guess I'm tired because I'm suddenly anemic again. My hematocrit this morning was a bit over 30, and I just gave enough blood away to drop a couple of points again.

I call Ruth, tell her to expect me in the office on Monday and to confirm Tuesday's surgery with the patient. I'm glad to have something to do while I wait this extra week.

Suddenly it's Wednesday again, my reprieve was so short, and we're back on the shuttle, this time later in the day, timing my arrival for the latest moment possible. No private room this time, my roommate is an elderly widow being evaluated for widespread metastatic breast cancer, and she can scarcely move because of pain from pathologic fractures in her vertebrae. That could be me, if this transplant doesn't work. She is a nice lady, and we enjoy each other's company.

The anesthesiologist comes by again for the anesthesia consent. Don't change a thing, I tell him, last week was perfect, anesthesia like it ought to be! He actually smiles. I didn't know he had it in him.

Ken comes by with the harvest consent, now it's February, so he's the attending of the month. Be sure you get enough, I tell him. Oh, we will, for sure. This batch will just be frozen untreated, just in case the treated marrow doesn't take. Ken has good news about the marrow they treated last week. The treatment was totally successful, they tested a small sample after they treated it and could find absolutely none of the cells they removed, the plasma cells, the B1 cells, the CALLA cells. Furthermore, all the plasma cells that were in the marrow before the treatment with the monoclonal antibodies stained normally, the immunoperoxidase stains showed that all the protein in the plasma cells was polyclonal in origin, not monoclonal, the latter being a sign of myeloma.

Does that mean I'm already cured? I don't need this transplant? Ken hesitates. No, I don't think so, I think you still need this transplant, the IgG is in the wrong proportion to the IgA and IgM, even though the numbers are in the normal range. But you are in a super remission. The brief flare of hope that there's a way out of this flickers and dies. I want the definitive treatment, the treatment to end all further treatment, I don't want to hang out and see if this remission turns into a cure. It never has before, and if I defer this treatment and the myeloma does come back, it may not be possible to get me into remission again. No, hit it when it's down, right now. Go for the cure.

I seem to be in more discomfort after this operation than last week, it's a little harder to move around. My pelvis must look like a colander. The anesthesia was perfect, I don't remember anything. My roommate has been moved to a private room, and I am alone. I'm wide awake, and actually I'd like to leave now, but I have to wait for the blood from my own marrow, just like last week.

In the early evening, after Jim has left for dinner with his sister, an attractive young man with a thick mop of curly hair wanders into my room after knocking tentatively at the open doorway. I've never seen him before, and he is casually dressed in jeans and a sweater. Must be a visitor looking for my roommate from yesterday, I surmise, and start to tell him that she was moved to another room. I'm looking for Dr. Thompson, he says. Yes, I say, that's me. He extends his hand. I'm a friend of Ken Anderson's, and he suggested I come by to see you. Oh? You see, he quickly explains, I had a bone marrow transplant six months ago, and Ken thought you'd like to talk to me. Boy, would I! Please sit down, tell me about it. I stare at him avidly—he looks so healthy, so well, so fit, all that hair!

I extract his story quickly: he's about ten years younger than I, also a doctor, although he's never practiced medicine since completing a residency in internal medicine five years ago, because that was when he discovered he had lymphoma, a malignancy of lymph glands involving cells related to the plasma cell malignancy I have. He tells me how he discovered his disease himself, driving down the Los Angeles freeway, feeling uncomfortable after a fast-food meal, reaching down to loosen his belt and feeling a greatly enlarged spleen. His diagnosis was quickly confirmed, and he has spent the last five years undergoing various treatments he has researched and, while well, supporting himself in business with his father. He is here now, all the way from California, for a six-month checkup with his doctor at Dana-Farber; in fact, he's meeting him for dinner tonight and has to leave soon.

I pepper him with questions about the transplant experience. How bad was it? Not so bad after the first two weeks, just boring after that. What was bad about the first two weeks? Well, it wasn't so much the nausea and vomiting, they control that pretty well with drugs, but you realize your mind is gone, squash rot; I think what happens is the radiation causes some cerebral edema, and you get an organic brain syndrome. You realize it when you try to read the newspaper and you read the same paragraph maybe ten times in a half hour and it still doesn't make sense to you. It's pretty upsetting when that happens, but just remember, it's temporary, it will go away after a couple of weeks. Also, everything is very hard to do, seems to take forever, simple things like taking a bath, eating breakfast.

What else? How was it after that? Boring mostly, I walked back and forth constantly, twelve steps one way, twelve steps back. I've arranged for a cross-country ski machine to be put in my room, I tell him. Why didn't I think of that? That would have been great!

He goes on, announces proudly that he is the only one who has ever gained weight in the transplant program, but they made such a big deal about the expected weight loss that he determined to force himself to eat, and he did, successfully gaining ten pounds overall. He had always been a prodigious eater anyway.

After he leaves, promising to call me after the first couple of weeks to see how I'm doing, I am elated. This won't be so bad. He looks wonderful! He survived! He's had no relapse! His marrow was treated with two of the same antibodies mine was treated with last week, and his marrow came back. He was in isolation for a month. I'm glad he warned me about the brain rot, and how temporary it is. I guess I won't get any productive work done for the first couple of weeks. I'm glad the cross-country machine will be there. That'll be more interesting than pacing the floor like a caged tiger.

We get out of the hospital late Friday morning. Heather and J will be arriving today sometime, and we plan an outing to a good restaurant with the four of us, plus Cox and Karen and Jim's sister Betsy. Another last supper. I feel like I've had a month of last suppers with all these postponements. I'll rest in the apartment, the pain from the second operation is making me tired. I take the pain medicine, no gold stars for bravery is what I tell my patients, use the pain pills if you have pain.

J arrives in the late afternoon, and he has brought all his favorite compact discs. For you, Mom, you can use them while you're in the hospital. I am incredibly touched by his thoughtfulness, his gift of love. Thank you, sweetie, but I might not want to listen to all of them, let's go over them. He plays various selections he thinks I'll especially like, and we select about three or four for me to keep. You take the rest back to school with you.

Heather's plane is delayed, and we go out for dinner without her, leaving word with the doorman to let her in. The umpteenth last supper is a nice dinner, everyone is in a festive mood, and I try to keep up with the mood, but it's a struggle, I have no appetite, I hurt, and I'm tired. It's a relief to get home, and we arrive just as Heather does, in a cab from the airport. The whole group troups upstairs to catch up with Heather, and I collapse on a sofa, watch from a great distance, will everyone to leave, soon, please. They do.

Ken wants me to check in at the hospital in the afternoon, but once all the tests are done, I can leave and come back after dinner. Great. Another last supper. Let's just have a quiet dinner downstairs in the dining room in our building.

Jim loads up most of my stuff, and we drag the schlepper to the hospital with us in the afternoon. Again a skeleton crew. I explain that the EKG and chest X ray don't need to be repeated, so we are escorted upstairs. The nurses are busy, we leave the bags in the nursing station, wait in the patients' lounge down the hall, and light up cigarettes. I've been smoking more than ever, I wonder if it will be hard to stop.

A young woman introduces herself as Karen, one of the nurses. She has a form for me to fill out, and we go through the questions about my health, my family, and she asks about the smoking. A temporary aberration, only the last few weeks, a way of coping with the stress. She explains, firmly, that smoking is absolutely forbidden in the room. I know, I know, I'll stop, I promise.

Do you wear contacts? Yes. You have to stop that, too, because of infection. But I have no glasses, haven't had any for over twenty years. I can't see without contact lenses, and no one can correct my vision with glasses, too much spectacle blur from wearing contacts. Ken said it might be okay to wear them. I don't think so, says Karen, but we can check it out next week with our ophthamologist. Meanwhile, you'll have to stop. I groan inwardly. Now I'll be locked in a room, and blind, too.

Karen explains that they want to draw some blood tests from one of my lines and the house officers need to do the admission history and physical, and then I'll be free to go and come back later, after dinner. Meanwhile, the nurses will wash all my belongings and put them in my room. Jim and I have already washed all the clothes and packed them in clean plastic bags as we were instructed to do last week by Felice. I won't go in the room until after dinner, because once I go in, I can't leave.

Karen pages the house staff to let them know I'm waiting to be done with them as soon as possible, and then she takes me into the utility room to draw the blood from one of my lines. This is one of the major advantages of having these lines, no more needle sticks. The intern and resident find me, and together we go off in search of an empty room where they can examine me for the official admission.

I find Jim in the patients' lounge, and we leave after ascertaining from the nurses that 10:30 tonight would not be too late to return. I spend the evening in the apartment with Jim and the children, and we have dinner downstairs in the formal dining room, just the four of us. The last last supper; my mood is desultory, sad, rebellious. J is letting us know how much he disapproves of our smoking, Jim is raising eyebrows at my desire for a second glass of wine, and we are all exhausted with the wait. After dinner, we settle back in the apartment, listen to music, and wait till the very last minute to leave.

I hug the children good-bye in the apartment, they'd rather see me in the hospital tomorrow than come over tonight. Jim and I walk in the cool night air, smoke a last cigarette, and I pitch my lighter and cigarettes into the wastebasket outside the building.

Karen greets us again. We sit in the patients' lounge as she explains the drill. Karen asks what I prefer to be called, how do I wish to be addressed while I'm here? I'm surprised by this, and consider for a moment. It's a pretty informal atmosphere around here, I tell her, just call me Cesca, but pronounce it right, Chess-ka, not Jessica. Okay, Karen responds. She leans forward now, eager and intense. How do you feel? Scared? I look at her. No, I feel confident. I think to myself, Yes, I am confident. I'll get through this without major infection, that's been my main concern, and

I've done my best to get ready. I look at Karen again, say I'm anxious to get this started and over with.

Karen explains to Jim that all small articles brought into the room have to be cleaned off and then placed in the pass-through closet, nothing comes through the door in your hands, which have just been washed and covered with sterile gloves after you've masked and gowned. This is reverse isolation, to keep outside bacteria away from me. It seems more ritualistic than complete to me, because there are no shoe covers or hair covers. Who's kidding whom; we wouldn't run an operating room like this.

I can enter the room in my street clothes, but only to go into the bathroom to shower with a special antiseptic soap and put on a whole set of clean clothes, and put all the things I'm wearing in a large paper bag, including my wig. My wig? What do you mean, my wig, can't I wear my wig? No, no one wears a wig here, they're not clean. Ken did not tell me about this, was he unaware that I'd mind a lot? What the hell, who am I going to see here, except my family, who have grown used to my bald head, and the staff, who take care of bald patients all the time?

By the time I've showered and changed into a set of clean surgical scrubs, Jim has completed his ablutions and entered the room and is standing awkwardly, gowned, masked, and holding his gloved hands in the air, not sure whether he can touch anything.

We look around the room. It's a standard single room. A large door to the corridor, with a window in it. I immediately draw the curtain, blocking the view into the room. I will not have people looking in at me, like a goldfish in a bowl. There are cupboards along the wall next to the door, and one set are double pass-through cupboards, where things are passed into the room from the outside. One side is to be closed at all times. There is a small closet, and a small counter built into this wall. Some of my things have been unpacked, but most are in brown paper shopping bags stacked neatly against the wall in the corner.

The bed is situated against the wall, so I could be easily seen from the window in the door if the curtain were left open. It is neatly made up, and there is a swinging attachment on the right that serves as a night table, which can be swung around close to the bed to make things easy to reach. On the wall opposite the bed is a large empty cork bulletin board, a good place for the photographs I've brought. The outside wall is small because the bathroom is on that wall, too, so the window to the outside world is at the end of a small alcove. Most of the space is occupied by a large stainless steel framework of shelves of the standard sort for utility and supply rooms. It has been abundantly stocked with intravenous paraphernalia, plastic cups, flatware, tea bags, sugar. The rest of the space is taken up by my cross-country ski machine, clean and new. A small refrigerator, just over knee-high, with a small freezer in it as well, nests against the wall opposite the bed.

Along the wall to the right and behind the bed is a large sink and mirror, and between the sink and the bed is a large white enamel doctor's-style scale. Karen points out the bottled water next to the sink, reminds me that I may not drink tap water, I must use the sterile water, even to clean my teeth.

In the central part of the room surrounding the bed are a single straight-backed chair, a curved easy chair with ottoman, and the typical narrow table for meals, which can be raised and lowered. In addition, there is a huge garbage-can-size wastebasket with plastic bag, and a portable toilet. This seems redundant to me, the bathroom being only steps away, and I wonder what they know that I don't that they assume I won't be able to walk to the toilet.

I've already noticed the toilet in the bathroom has little plastic pots that sit in it, obviously for my use, so that both urine and stool can be measured before flushing away. No privacy at all here.

Jim and I spend about an hour unpacking, finding homes for things, and I make the space my own by arranging photographs on the bulletin board, small objects next to the bed, in addition to the radio and portable compact disc player. Finally, Jim leaves me, we hug surreptitiously, suspecting this is against the rules, too.

A technician arrives with a portable X-ray machine, they can't find my recent chest X rays from last week at the other hospital and want to take one now, "for baseline." "Baseline" is a term used to establish a starting point for later comparison, as in, what does this chest look like on the picture we get here, shooting at the patient standing in the doorway with her back to the machine, clutching a large cold X-ray plate to her chest, taking a deep breath, and holding it? What it looks like is nothing, evidently, because the technician is back in about a half hour, saying the picture is technically inadequate, she wants to shoot another. Forget it, I say, you've had your chance, and I have no reason to suspect you'll get it right this time either, and I will be getting enough radiation for a lifetime this week, I won't take anymore. Okay, she shrugs, glad to roll her machine away. I am annoyed that I even consented to the first X ray, I should have realized there are always problems with late night portables. I should have postponed it till tomorrow and asked Ken if I really had to have it, now I've been blasted to no purpose at all. I resolve to object strenuously to any further X rays shot in the doorway.

SUNDAY, FEBRUARY 8, 1987

First day of treatment for me, first day in the hospital, but the protocol counts this as day minus-5, five days till I get my treated marrow, the transplant, and then we start counting survival days, or days to engraftment. In these five days I get blasted. First the intravenous Alkeran, then the radiation.

When the nurse comes in, I ask her what all the catheter equipment is for, stacked neatly near my bed. She explains that the chemo will involve bladder irrigation. I remember that unpleasantness from my last consolidation round, and I remember, too, that Ken had told me, when I asked, that no bladder irrigation was required for the Alkeran. I tell her it is my understanding that this is for Cytoxan therapy, not Alkeran, and we will not do it until she double-checks with Dr. Anderson and I talk to him too. A little later, she removes all the offending equipment, tells me I am right. I am relieved. That bladder irrigation was no fun last time.

The nurse runs my bath, adds pink antiseptic solution that bubbles up wildly, explains this is a daily ritual after breakfast. How about a shower? No, that was okay last night, but now we don't want you to wash in tap water, it's not as clean as this special bubble bath, with soap generally used for preop scrubbing. I don't use this soap when I scrub for the OR, because it leaves a thin oily residue on my hands that gets on my contact lenses and blurs them like the diesel residue on a car's windshield. I guess that doesn't matter now that I can't wear my contacts. The tub is small, on a diagonal, I can barely stretch my legs out straight, even sitting up and leaning back, but the water is hot and the bubbles are fun, cool against my skin.

After my bath I dive into my white terry cloth robe and wait for my nurse to return to do the dressings on my lines, something we'll do every day here. She peels off the plastic covering, and I wince. This is getting harder and harder, my skin is reacting to the plastic, blistering and red. This hurts, but what we're both concerned about is the potential for infection if my skin breaks down. She finds a different sticky plastic, maybe I won't react to that one so much.

Heather and J come over with Jim in the morning, before the chemo starts. J has to go back to school, but at least he can see me settled and cheerful in my room, he will have a mental image of this room when he talks to me later. Both children study their photographs on the corkboard, a sequence covering the years since their birth. It seems like that's when I started taking and saving pictures, and most of the pictures have one or both of the children and Jim in them. A few have me, a different me, smiling and healthy, with hair, did I ever look like that? The children leave before the chemo starts. I urge them to call me often, daily even. They seem anxious to leave. This is not a comfortable place to be, all masked and gowned, afraid to touch anything.

Like last time, they give me intravenous hydration before starting the actual drug, around noon this time. I negotiate the anti-emetic drugs with the nurse, start off with the marijuana pills I brought from New York, and get so stoned I scarcely notice the day going by. Jim spends the day with me, he plans to be here all week for the treatment and the transplant. I am only vaguely aware he's here. He's watching TV, but I don't bother. I can't see the screen up on the wall, even if I could keep my eyes open.

By suppertime, I start vomiting. No one is surprised. My nurse points out that the marijuana pills may not stay down, would I try some of their IV stuff? You bet, give it your best shot. I wake fitfully to vomit some more through the night.

The second round of Alkeran isn't quite as bad. I use both intravenous sedation and the marijuana for nausea control, and it's a bit better. Still stoned, though, and unpleasantly so. I hope this gets better tomorrow: just radiation, no chemotherapy.

Today I get my eyes tested for real glasses; everyone agrees my lenses could be a real disaster. With no protective white cells and most likely diminished tears because of the radiation, a common complaint following radiation therapy, I'd really be set up for an eye infection. Ken has persuaded his eye guy to come over to the hospital to refract me for glasses. He's a very nice man, understands the problem of spectacle blur after years of contact lenses, especially poorly fitted ones, as mine probably were, and explains that my eyes will gradually assume their regular shape as they are no longer molded by my lenses, and he will have to readjust the prescription every month or so until my eyes stabilize. He's brought a selection of frames, too, and I try a few on. I think I like big, tortoiseshell frames, what do you think, Jim? What looks good with a bald head? I must be stoned if I think this is funny.

My nurse rushes me through breakfast, which is now coffee and little else, and into a hospital gown and robe for my trip to radiation therapy. The ambulance will be here soon. Yes, I will be delivered two blocks away by ambulance. The ambulance attendants arrive, are masked, gowned, and gloved. I am allowed to walk through the door, to lie on the stretcher and get wrapped from head to toe in blankets. A towel is wrapped around my head, and I am given a mask as well. I must look like E.T.

Surrounded by a nurse, Jim, Heather, and two ambulance attendants, IV bags dangling from poles, I get pushed along on the stretcher. One ambulance attendant has the job of clearing the halls, and he walks about twenty feet ahead, waving people out of the way, asking them to leave until we pass by, emptying elevators, and making a complete spectacle of our little procession. The outside air is cool, despite the infrared lighting in the ambulance bay. The drive is short, it doesn't take long to go two blocks, and then the whole performance is repeated, sweeping curious onlookers away, like Moses and the Red Sea. The waiting room for radiation therapy has been cleared of other patients, and I am swept immediately into the treatment room and transferred to the table.

Not a table, really, it's a very tight hammock, so tight it's flat, but made of a very thin nylon type of material. It has to be thin, the technician explains, because this machine is so advanced it delivers radiation from two directions at once, top and bottom, so the rads are delivered in half the time and there is no need to turn me. She sets about taping the lead protectors on my chest, front and back. They look like thin lead fish. She outlines the shields on my skin with magenta-colored marker for quicker placement next time. I remember seeing radiation patients marked up with that color before, and the recollection depresses me. Yes, I'm one of them.

My watch and ring are removed and handed to Jim for safekeeping. Out of my blankets for several minutes now, I complain of the cold. The technician gives me one sheet, says any more covering would interfere with the radiation dose. Everyone evacuates, and the machine is revved up. I lie motionless, the twenty minutes passes rapidly, I picture all my plasma cells getting zapped, especially the myeloma cells, no we don't want to leave even one, no matter where they are, in or out of the marrow.

The trip back to my room is another charade, but I'm cold and tired now and grateful to be able to get back to my room quickly. I just want to get in bed and curl up under the covers. No chance. It's decontamination time, every time I come back from radiation I have to take a bath in the antiseptic soap, just in case I got contaminated in the radiation room.

The days orient themselves around the trips outside, the radiation treatment. Nausea signals the need for more medication, which is readily available, and I waft in and out of naps. I am not surprised I feel bad, actually I am relieved it's not as bad as I expected. By Thursday afternoon I've completed six trips to radiation, two a day. My treatment is complete.

Ken arrives at suppertime, smiling broadly and carrying a small clear plastic bag with a pale pink liquid in it. He holds it up, Here's your transplant. I am amazed at how small it is, it looks like four ounces, at best six ounces. This is going to replace my bone marrow? It feels like magic. Ken and the nurse hook it up to my IV, and we watch it drip in. What day is today, Ken asks, February 12? Yes. Your new birthday! Great, Lincoln and me; at least I'm still Aquarius.

What's that smell? I ask. Ken smiles. We use some DMSO, a solvent, to freeze the marrow, and it smells like very strong garlic. I reek. How long is this going to last? Probably till tomorrow. I look at Jim and Ken. I don't know how you can stand it. They don't seem to mind. The transfusion of my treated marrow is complete, and Ken gives me the bag somewhat ceremoniously. I hand it to Jim, tell him to pin it to the corkboard so I can see it. My new glasses have been delivered, and I can see across the room now.

The chemoradiotherapy is finished, and I have my treated marrow. Now we wait, wait for the counts to go down, wait for something bad to happen, wait for the counts to come back, wait till I can get out of here. I am way past the point of no return.

Jim stays a week longer than he had planned, because a few days after the transplant, I am feeling worse and worse, instead of better. My skin is burned, my throat hurts so much I can't swallow, and I feel tired, bone-deep tired. Jim learns from the nurse that this is entirely predictable and will get worse, so he decides to spend another week in Boston. I am glad he is here, look forward to his arrival every morning, am comforted by his presence, reading and watching TV by my bedside. I miss him when he goes out to meals. We don't talk much; I can't focus outward at all, consumed as I am by a constant awareness of how lousy I feel. The nurse is right, it does get worse, the nausea and vomiting get worse instead of better. For about a week I make no pretense of even trying fluids, and I stay on round-the-clock anti-emetics, marijuana in the daytime, Ativan at night.

After Jim returns to New York, my mother starts to spend Tuesday through Saturday in our apartment and sits with me during the day and into the evening. I don't know how she can stand it, I am not very good company at all. I appreciate her being there, but I have no energy to talk. She brings books, tapes, books-on-tape, and all sorts of amusing clippings. I am not amused, indeed, I am resolutely unamusable. I don't care what Norman Cousins says about curing yourself with laughter, my sense of humor is gone. Well, almost. One day I have an insight that I think is very funny and laugh uproariously when I tell Ken about it: Convalescence, I announce importantly, is no fun when you're not feeling well.

Jim flies up from New York on Fridays in the late afternoon and takes my mother out to dinner after visiting for a while, returns afterward. My mother returns to Litchfield Saturday mornings, and Jim spends the weekend sitting with me, watching TV. He usually arrives in time for a Saturday-morning educational show with cartoons on the theory of relativity. I find myself watching these cartoons of Albert Einstein traveling at the speed of light, and I never seem to get it, instead I'm struggling with more nausea. The weekends are worse somehow, I don't know why, the rhythm of the weekday is not there, the staff is different, I don't trust the weekend laboratory data to be as accurate, and most weekends I am trying to wean myself away from the mind-blowing medicine, feeling that maybe the last couple of days have been a bit better, I can do without so much stuff. Not for long, and not without getting into a whole vitiating round of uncontrollable vomiting again. Somehow Jim gets to be here when I'm at my worst, this must be horrible for him.

Jim takes the Sunday night shuttle back, and I face the

prospect of being alone in Boston till Tuesday afternoon, when my mother arrives again. Jim calls to let me know he arrived safely and usually catches me on the phone again in the daytime, after my counts are ready. I don't know what's worse for him, being cooped up with me in mask and gown all day, knowing that I'm okay but feeling miserable, or being able to get his mind off this at work, but not knowing if I'm okay.

The days start to be the same. To be asleep is so wonderful, I prolong it as long as possible, way past my normal six A.M. rising. I try to sleep, scrunched under the covers till the house staff makes morning rounds. Luckily, these are medical house officers, not ones to make dawn rounds, as I used to on my surgical rotations. They usually arrive in my room between eight and nine A.M. They are masked and gowned, of course, and change so often I can't keep track of their names. Two or three of them listen to my chest and heart at the same time, one of them peers at my throat with a flashlight and asks me how I am, and we have a brief discussion. This is a ritual, I know. The intern's job is to write a note every day in my chart, and he has to have something to say, he has to keep track of my numbers, and he should be on top of things if they start going bad. We both know Ken is my doctor. Every time the house officers leave, they ask if there is any thing they can do for me. I say no, thank you. What I want to say is stop asking me if there is anything you can do for me! Don't treat me like you think I'm dying! When I was a house officer, we used to ask only the dying patients if there was anything we could do for them. Every time I hear the question, I hear their assessment of my situation—diagnosis: multiple myeloma; prognosis: death.

Soon after the departure of the house staff, my nurse of the day comes in to draw blood from my line, several tubes a day. It's good I have two lines, the one on the right won't draw. Although I would like to prolong the night a while longer, I really can't anymore. It's bath time, and they want to change my sheets. Forget breakfast, I've stopped eating. I dawdle in the tub, swish the water around, absorb the heat, note the radiation-induced changes in my skin, first as overall deep sunburn, then an all-over tan, slightly yellowish.

Out of the tub and into my terry cloth robe, I wait for my nurse to do the daily dressing change on my two lines. The skin blistering prevents the use of the sticky stuff, so I invent an unusual dressing, lots of sterile surgical pads tucked into my bra, which sounds simple but is difficult to execute and requires speed, agility, and persistence on the part of my nurse and myself to avoid contaminating one or both lines.

The nurse usually asks if I've done my mouth care. We both know I won't follow their ritual, and they are hoping for some minimal cooperation on my part. There is an elaborate regimen I am supposed to follow four times a day, to make up for not being able to brush my teeth with a regular toothbrush or to floss, forbidden because of the likelihood of bleeding and possibly sending mouth bacteria into my bloodstream. Instead, they have giant Q-Tips to scrub my gums and teeth with, using hydrogen peroxide, then they want me to suck on an antifungal vaginal suppository and swish with some foul-tasting stuff. I find it's guaranteed to induce forceful vomiting. No way. I work out my own thing, a gauze pad dipped in sterile water and wrapped around my index finger, with which I gently scrub the gunk. If I'm very, very careful, it doesn't make me gag and vomit. I do this once a day, occasionally twice. The nurses do not approve, mutter darkly about terrible mouth infections I'll get. I don't care, I say to myself, nothing's worse than vomiting.

I settle into my clean sheets and watch TV or listen to music. At first I tune into Oprah Winfrey, find it amusing, but soon the shows are too sad, dealing with child abuse, wife battering; I cannot cope with so much sorrow, especially the phone calls. It's easier to listen to the radio, "lite" music, only slightly better than elevator music, but not demanding. I listen and drift, wait till the mail arrives around eleven. My tapes and compact discs are too complex to attend to, much less start and stop. Some of the ones I listen to initially become associated with the violent nausea and vomiting I experienced in the first few days, and because I'm constantly on the brink of barfing again, I avoid them. Friends have sent me new tapes and compact discs of operas and other treasured music, and I am reluctant to listen to them, not wanting to get Verdi associated with this terrible malaise.

I get several phone calls in the morning. These perk me up, I can mobilize for a phone call. Heather calls every day. J doesn't call as often, but I think they check in with each other constantly. Jim calls. My mother calls. Friends call. We generally talk briefly about how I'm doing. I am told so often that I sound better than I did last time that I begin to think I must sound strange indeed. Certainly it is hard to enunciate with a dry mouth, and I haven't had any saliva for days. A radiation effect, apt to last weeks or months. When I feel moderately decent, I try to change the topic to focus on what's happening in my caller's life. I'd much rather hear about that, it takes me out of where I am now. Also, it's easier to listen than to talk for the several weeks of sore throat and mouth pain. Later these same friends will tell me that I had trouble remembering what they told me over the space of only two or three minutes.

Mail is delivered soon after eleven. My brother Reto's wife sends me a funny card a day. So does my older sister, who, despite her vacation, has arranged to have cards mailed to me daily. In addition to those, there are usually one or two letters a day from colleagues who have received my letter and are writing to express sympathy, to wish me well. These letters are always moving, often profoundly so. Every couple of days I respond to the collection of letters I have, thank each person for thinking of me, tell them that although I feel lousy, everything is going very well, no infection or other bad stuff.

Sometime after the mail is delivered, I call out to the desk and ask what my counts are today. My nurse then comes in with the numbers scribbled on a scrap of paper, and I write it down on the calendar on the corkboard opposite me. When my platelets are under 20,000 or my hematocrit below 28, I know I'll be getting a transfusion later.

The white count settles to nothing and stays that way for days and days. This is the scary part. I am at the most-vulnerable-to-infection stage now, with no immune system of my own to fight it. This means, of course, that the chemoradiotherapy has done what it was supposed to do: destroy my marrow and, we hope, the cancer with it. Now I need my transplanted cells to come back, to show that the marrow transplant has taken, has engrafted. If my white count doesn't show an increase by at most three weeks after the transplant, there's that second, untreated marrow waiting to be used to rescue me, the fail-safe marrow that would save my life for now but would give me back the myeloma cells. So far so good, though, I have no signs of infection and am getting by with no immune system.

After what feels like ages, my white count begins to show an increase, meaning engraftment of the transplant, around post-transplant day 13, February 25. The marrow has taken! That's a big relief, we won't have to rescue me with untreated marrow, that second harvest of bone marrow can remain on ice in perpetuity. I am regenerating a treated marrow, one with none of the malignant myeloma cells in it. If the chemoradiation therapy really did destroy the diseased cells, every single one, then I'm cured now, all I have to do is survive. But 200 white cells, almost none of them polys, the bacteria fighters, leaves me a long way from getting out of here.

The cross-country ski machine stands idle, mocking me for my naive faith that I could stay in shape while confined in a small room. What nonsense! I can barely walk to the bathroom, pushing my IV pump. I used the machine a couple of times, in that small window of time after the immediate nausea of chemoradiotherapy subsided and before the sore throat and the drop in my counts, the return of inexplicable nausea and vomiting. The fatigue I am experiencing is relentless. I don't understand it, but it's there, pressing me back into my bed like extra gravity. Sitting up in the chair is out of the question, and after the second week I stop trying. The physical therapist comes by with a list of exercises she's willing to show me. I look at her balefully, tell her I feel terrible, and now is not a good time. If I feel better, I'll call her, I say. I never do.

Occasionally I try a lunch tray, chicken noodle soup or chicken rice. The smell of food is truly nauseating to me in my present state of constant nausea. My food trays have to be wrapped in sterile bags. Unfortunately, these bags also trap the smell of the food and because the trays, for sterility's sake, cannot be unwrapped until they are placed in my room, all the food fumes are released in one fell swoop for me to gag over. The olfactory blast is usually enough to extinguish any semblance of appetite I had entertained, and the tray goes untouched.

Hunger is rarely a problem. Sometimes I recognize a real hunger, especially early in the morning, around four A.M., when my night nurse comes in to fuss with my IV and wakes me up, but it's hard to feel hungry and nauseated at the same time, and the nausea always wins. I get on the scales daily, as ordered, and note that I'm losing about a quarter to a half kilo a day. No one else is worried about this, evidently it's totally expected.

I try the soaps in the afternoon once or twice, but somehow I can't follow them. What with dozing off a little or getting sidetracked with a phone call for a few minutes, I don't know when one show stops and another begins, so I'm getting all the plots confused. I remember what that guy who talked to me about his transplant said about losing brain power. My dementia seems to be lasting a lot longer than two weeks, I really haven't cleared my head at all. Reading novels is too hard. I am stuck in the middle of a submarine chase, have read one page over and over, and still I don't get it.

It gets dark early, and the official beginning of the evening for me is Phil Donahue at four. Good, sleep will come soon. Then it's Archie Bunker and Edith during the hospital dinnertime, two shows from five to six, and then the news. "McNeil-Lehrer" is on earlier in Boston than in New York and I watch avidly, between phone calls and the evening rounds of the attending staff, Ken in February, Jerry Ritz and Linda Bosserman in March. Ken stops by every evening anyway, even when he is not the official attending responsible for my day-to-day care.

Ken is always cheerful, emphasizes how well I'm doing, voices his concern that today hasn't been "a good day," maybe tomorrow will be a good day. I don't know what a good day would be. Would it be no nausea, no vomiting, no need for drugs that leave me unpleasantly stoned, no sore throat, no burning epigastric pain, no fatigue, no dry mouth, no loss of taste? Look at the bright side, you have hardly any fever, isn't that great? Yeah, that's great. How's the man down the hall? He's having a hard time, got a widespread fungus infection from an ingrown toenail, now has fungus in his eye, may lose his eye. Yes, things sure could be worse, I could be as sick as I feel.

As the weeks go by and the appropriate time for the nausea and vomiting to abate is long past, I complain that the antibiotics are making me feel worse. Every time they are hung, I feel more nausea and vomiting. Ken insists we need them, I have either no white cells or so few that I still need the antibiotics. But the dose is so high, especially the gentamicin, 150 milligrams three times a day, that's twice the dose I used to use on very sick patients. I'm worried about the side effects of hearing loss and kidney damage gentamicin is known to induce in high dose. Ken points out that my blood levels of gentamicin are in the safe range, and my BUN and creatinine, simple blood tests of kidney function, are quite low. Of course they're low, they depend on protein metabolism, and I haven't eaten in weeks. I'm starving and the only protein I'm getting is my own muscle mass, and here I stretch out my newly wasted arm, which is fast disappearing. See? Yes, but I think you're doing okay, and you ought to stay on the antibiotics.

How about TPN, total parenteral nutrition? It would be possible to feed me enough calories to stop my weight loss via the IV, do you think we ought to consider that? I still can't eat. It hurts going down, and when I get it down, it sits there, and I get more and more nauseated and feel like I've had way too much to eat, and then I usually throw it up. Ken admits to being puzzled by my inability to eat and keep food down, this usually lasts only ten to fourteen days, and he can only surmise that it's the combination of the huge dose of Alkeran and the radiation that none of their other patients has ever had before that accounts for this prolonged food intolerance. But as far as TPN is concerned, they have done studies on whether TPN helps or not, and they've concluded that it increases the risk of infection a little, because of the high sugar concentration in the lines, which represents an excellent medium for bacterial growth. So they'd rather hold off. I concede that although I am weak and exhausted all the time, I am far from underweight as yet.

No evening is complete without a call from my friend who was a resident with me at the Hospital for Special Surgery. He calls every night between six and nine, without fail. Sometimes we talk for less than a minute, sometimes for fifteen or twenty minutes, depending on how I feel. It's always good to hear from him.

Nights are the worst and best time. Unconsciousness is best, but I usually can't get through the night without waking several times. Light filters in through the window in the door from the outside hallway. Most of the night nurses are men working a ten- or twelve-hour shift. Their main job is hanging my medicines, and I get antibiotics and antiviral medicine around the clock, so that they have to fuss with my IV at ten P.M., two A.M., four A.M., and although they try to be quiet and use a small flashlight, I'm not asleep deeply enough to sleep through it. I usually ask for Ativan, they hang it in my other line, and I slip into sleep again, duck under the nausea that wells up with wakefulness.

Falling-asleep time is the best time to use imagery, and every night I have three or four chances to imagine my myeloma cells exploding, to visualize the abnormal protein disappearing, turning the upward spike in the tracing of my protein level to a downward-pointing dimple in an otherwise normal curve, as if that entire population of protein were removed completely. For some reason, all my imaging is directed to eradicating my disease. I never consider imagining being without nausea; this is only a symptom, a subjective problem, not the real problem that we are getting rid of here.

I get the feeling that some of the nurses think I'm vomiting for attention, that it's psychological, not physical. They send in a nurse to teach me some relaxation techniques. I'm supposed to close my eyes and imagine I'm on a beautiful beach, listening to the water coming in and out. Not a chance. I throw up again, I feel discouraged and helpless, sob hysterically while Jim drapes a cool wet washcloth on my bald head, oddly soothing. I'm losing it totally now, I'm never going to get out of here if I can't eat, no matter what my counts are, and it's been five weeks in here and still I can't keep two meals in a row down! Jim is reassuring, points to the computer printout he's made of my improving white counts, which has the new place of honor on the corkboard, and lets me know that eventually I will get out of here. It doesn't seem real to me. Jim is literally holding me together, not only physically, with his arms around me, but emotionally as well, lending me his conviction that I will make it through when I have lost hope.

Jerry Ritz and Linda Bosserman, the attendings for March, start giving me pep talks, tell me I should be up and around more, out of bed in a chair more, and imply that my laziness is the cause of my nausea and malaise. They couldn't be more wrong. I know me, and I know that if I felt better I would be doing more. I think about their unfeeling, blame-the-victim attitude, and recall with some remorse how many times I've laid that trip on one of my patients, a little old lady struggling with the trauma of hip fracture surgery, for instance. Never again.

The white count starts to come up but hangs out at a low level, too low to stop the antibiotics, too low to go home. Jerry and Linda step up their campaign to get me thinking about leaving the hospital. What's the use of thinking about it, will you let me leave if I can't keep food down? Still, you have to make plans, where will you stay, who's going to take care of you? I have an apartment nearby, and if Jim can't take care of me, I'm sure there's a home health agency that can send someone in. That's not the problem, the problem is I can't even hydrate myself yet, and my white count is too low by your criteria for me to come off the antibiotics, so let's not even talk about it, let's not get my hopes up.

By the middle of March the white cells take a leap from the plateau of 700 cells to 1700, or 1.7, and this is sustained for a couple of days. One of my Hickman catheters is removed by Chip Moore at the request of the medical team, who are worried that it may be infected because it is not drawing blood. Actually it hasn't been drawing blood since I went into the hospital, but never mind. Chip doesn't like to remove a good line before its time, but he does come over after a few requests and removes the line with some local anesthetic and much pulling and tugging. Those lines really do scar into the velcro cuff right under the skin. No fever develops after pulling the line, and the white count stays up at 1.7.

We are in the home stretch, and to convince me that this is so, the antibiotics are discontinued on March 20, thirty-five days after the transplant. I've been on high-dose intravenous antibiotics for thirty days. I've had a few low-grade fevers, but nothing much in the infectious disease category. I guess they worked. Good, now I don't have those lousy antibiotics making me sick anymore. I expect to feel better. I don't.

We're not making much progress, I complain to the doctors, the nurses, all who will listen. I persuade them to unhook my intravenous in the daytime, hoping that if I'm not given intravenous fluids I might get thirsty enough to try to get some wet stuff down. The nurses are avid in detailing how many ounces I drink all through the day. It's not enough, they have to crank up the fluids at night so I don't get dehydrated, but each day I do take in a little bit more.

Linda and Jerry are now suggesting other food and drink I might try, and suggest a milkshake. Are you sure? A real milkshake? Not some bottled evaporated milk thing that tastes terrible? Sure, the kitchen will make it up for you. It's Friday night, Jim is already there, and we are both excited at this new liberty. As soon as we can, I order the milkshake, preferably chocolate, but strawberry's okay too. Sorry, kitchen is closed now, but they'll send you one in the morning.

Morning comes, and no milkshake. Finally it comes, and it's some canned, prepared food. Forget it, this is not what we were talking about. Sorry, it's the only kind of milkshake you can have on the cooked-food diet. It doesn't matter much, I'm throwing up again anyway, probably would have tossed a real milkshake as well.

Jerry and Linda come by again in the evening. The milkshake was a bust, it isn't on the diet. How about some fruit? You mean an orange or a banana? Sure. Are you sure I can have that? Oh, yes. They leave, I order the orange and the banana. Word filters back in a while. Sorry, the doctors have left, and fresh orange and banana are not on the cooked-food diet, and we can't send it up.

By now I am really angry. Two days in a row now these loony-tunes have come in all smiles and encouragement, offering food that actually appeals to me, and leave without writing the necessary order, in fact, seem so out of it that they don't even know what food is and is not on the diet. I resolve to stop discussing anything with them anymore, they obviously don't know what they are doing. Tomorrow I will tell them to get lost when they ask how I'm doing. Jim has been there at each discussion and is as perplexed as I am.

On Sunday afternoon, Jerry and Linda walk in all smiles. Before I can tell them to get out of my room, as we have nothing to discuss, Jerry announces that I am no longer on isolation, I can leave my room, and I can eat whatever I want. As soon as I demonstrate that I can keep enough fluid down without IV hydration at night, I can leave the hospital. I am stunned, and so is Jim. But my counts aren't so hot, I point out with stubborn pessimism. What about that famous requirement that the polys have to count up to 500? Mine are only about 250 to 300, only 16 percent of my overall white count. Jerry responds that he thinks they'll come up quickly, maybe even faster if I mobilize and walk outside the room a bit, and eat better. And stop being a slug, he means.

I do want to get out of the room, but not as a baldy. Jim makes a trip back to the apartment to get my wig. I put on my hair and peer at myself in the mirror through my large tortoiseshell glasses. I certainly look better, no longer like those pictures of the Chernobyl disaster victims I saw in *Life* magazine last summer, which is what I've been seeing in the mirror every day for weeks. But I look different, too. Hair on my head accentuates the hollows in my face, both along my temples and below my cheekbones.

The nurses make me put on a mask, for my protection against ambient germs. The mask smells, and I feel very self-conscious wearing it, as if I were wearing a sign, HEY, EVERYBODY, I'M REALLY SICK. My legs are rubbery, even tremulous, and I find I am staring at my feet, as if they wouldn't function without a visual assist. We make it all around the floor, and I return to my bed exhausted but elated. We'll do that again as soon as I can. My universe has suddenly expanded. It's been forty-three days in isolation in that room.

We leave the door open, the curtain pulled back, and the nurses come and go without the yellow gowns, masks, and gloves. I recognize them after a moment's hesitation, relying on movement and voice—their faces are totally new to me, and their bodies look different without the gowns.

A tray is carried in, no plastic wrap. A ham sandwich, milk, and red grapes. No disgusting smell of steamed food. The sandwich is good, on soft white bread with mayonaise and lettuce. I eat about half of it, it's tasty but very difficult to chew. The radiation therapy has left me with almost no saliva, and even with frequent sips of milk, food sticks to my teeth, it is a big effort to swallow. The grapes are wet and crunchy, much easier to eat.

Jim and I go for another walk around the floor before he has to return to New York. It's Sunday night again. We plan for the coming week: Jerry Ritz thinks I'll be able to leave on Tuesday, Jim will fly back then and stay with me for as long as it takes to get the okay to return to New York, possibly as much as two weeks. J is at home and may want to come up to Boston, now that he's over the strep throat he developed out in Utah skiing with friends over his vacation. He has stayed in New York to avoid infecting me. Heather could have come to Boston also for a few days of her spring vacation, but stayed away because of a cold as well, and now she's back in Ohio.

After Jim leaves, I sit in my room with the door open, and the woman in the room next to me drops by for a visit. She's a woman about my age, wearing the hospital bathrobe and a pale blue turban. I can see from the small part of her uncovered hair near her forehead that she has about a half inch of regrowing hair. Like jail inmates we compare notes: What're you in for? She's in for metastatic ovarian cancer. I maintain a bland, curious attitude but inwardly groan, Oh, no, and she seems so nice, mentally cringing at the devastatingly poor prognosis for her disease. She's going to get "rescued" with her own marrow tomorrow, she's just had very high doses of chemotherapy and her counts are way down, but her own marrow was harvested for this purpose, and tomorrow she'll probably get it back. She is on the solid-tumor marrow transplant service, a different group of researchers, and their protocol is different, no isolation because they have not attempted to eradicate the bone marrow and the patients are not nearly as compromised as patients with diseases of the bone marrow. She has children, too, of elementary school age, and we talk for a bit about how they've adjusted to her absence, so much harder for younger children. She brings me into her room to show me pictures her children have drawn for her, and I am almost in tears, remembering when Heather and J used to draw pictures like that, suddenly grateful I had so much time with them. This woman probably will not be so lucky. I feel a sudden need to extricate myself from getting to know her any better, it's too sad for me to cope with, I'm losing my resilience, my distance.

Late Sunday evening Ken comes by, and although he already knew of my "graduation" from isolation, he is surprised and delighted by my apparent restoration to health when he sees me sitting up in my chair, with my wig on, doing needlepoint. When he leaves, I walk him to the elevator. We are both very pleased, the worst is behind me.

On Monday I walk around the floor several times, "forgetting" my mask as often as I can get away with it. I make a concerted effort to take in enough fluid to prove I can make it on my own out there in the real world, and get into a ham sandwich rut—that first one was so good, I can't think of anything I'd rather have. The kitchen is happy to comply.

My neighbor from next door drops by for a visit, and as we talk I smell a familiar, unpleasant odor I can't identify until she tells me she recently got her transplant. Of course, the DMSO! That horrible garlic smell! I am amazed that on the protocol she's on she can wander around from room to room, but she's getting this to boost her recovery from chemotherapy, which was not designed to totally destroy her marrow, and didn't. We chat a little longer, then I plead exhaustion, and I tell her I have to rest up for my big day tomorrow, getting out of here.

TUESDAY, MARCH 24, 1987

Jim calls me early Tuesday morning. A disaster at the office, today of all days. All the word processing files for the last three years at the entire agency have been erased inadvertently, just disappeared in a technical glitch. He can't leave yet, there's hope that the computer company will be able to retrieve the information from the disc. He sounds distraught, and the last thing I want is for him to be worried about fetching me. J can come up here and get me. Do you think so? Jim asks. Sure, he was going to come up anyway, he can handle it. But I have all the cash, he doesn't have enough to get up there. I'll talk to him and we'll figure it out and let you know.

I wake J up, he has a tendency to stay up all night on

vacations and sleep most of the day, living on the other side of the clock. I explain about the disaster at the office, Dad can't come up, you have to come get me out of here. I think J is pleased to do this, because he quickly suggests that he can go to his bank and withdraw enough cash, and he'll come up to Boston right away. I tell him to go to the apartment here before coming to the hospital, because I need suitcases to pack into and clothes to wear. J writes down what he needs to pick up. See you soon, Mom.

The morning passes slowly, and I spend some time putting things in shopping bags, but packing is arduous— actually, just standing up is the hard part, and I sit down frequently to rest. J finally arrives with my clothes, and I soon discover he has forgotten to pack my pants. J, I think you better go back to the apartment and get my pants so I can get dressed. Oops, sorry, Mom. I am exasperated by his absentmindedness, and at the same time proud to see him so grown-up at sixteen that he can fly up to a strange city to come retrieve me from the hospital and take care of me till Jim can get here.

I try to pack some more, but am too exhausted. When J gets back, I get him to throw everything in the duffel bags while I sit and watch. One of my regular day nurses talks to J about my fatigue, says, Your mother is going to be very tired, she will have to take frequent naps, and this is normal, it will only gradually go away. J just looks at her, wide-eyed and solemn.

I retreat to the bathroom to get dressed. My clothes are very loose, but not that loose. I am a little disappointed, I think they should be falling off me after close to a thirty-pound weight loss in six weeks. Just getting dressed is a big effort, and I sit down to rest again. We are just about ready to go. The nurse offers a wheelchair to get me downstairs, where we'll call a cab. I jut my chin out stubbornly, no way, I'm leaving on my own two legs, thanks.

I wait on the sofa by the front door of the hospital while J calls a cab. It takes a long ten or fifteen minutes before the cab is there, amazing how long it seems when just sitting upright requires great strength. The cabdriver is none too pleased at such a short ride but delivers us to the door of our apartment house. It's a long way to our apartment, and by the time I get there I am totally spent and flop down on the sofa near the telephone.

I look out the window. It's a beautiful sunny crisp day, my first chance to be outside since February 7, and I didn't even notice the fresh air. I am out of the hospital, I survived, how come I don't feel happy? How come I feel like crying again? Because you feel like shit, that's why, and you're not sure that you haven't lost your health forever.

I call Jim, let him know we are ensconced in the apartment and will be fine together till he can come up. Take as long as you need to clear up the problem down there, J is here and can take care of me just fine. J smiles from across the room with some pride. Jim says it should be cleared up by tomorrow afternoon. Fine, J can take me back to the hospital in the morning for my clinic appointment, Ken wants to check my platelets before I get the second line pulled tomorrow afternoon at Chip Moore's office. If my platelet count is borderline I'll have to get a transfusion.

WEDNESDAY, MARCH 25 TO SATURDAY, APRIL 4, 1987

We order a cab in the morning, and J supports my arm as we walk slowly into the hospital. The role reversal is touching; I think of J as a toddler, when I gripped his chubby hand to cross the street, and now my man-size child is walking me. I am directed to the blood-drawing area, where we sit and wait for about ten minutes, not a long time, but an eternity to me, because sitting upright in a straight-backed chair is an enormous effort. Finally the nurse draws the blood from my arm after I refuse a needle stick in my finger. She doesn't have the necessary equipment or training to draw from the indwelling catheter that will be removed later today. She tells me to go on over to the adult clinic area to wait for the results.

By the time J walks me slowly over to the adult clinic, I feel so weak and dizzy I think I'm going to keel over. I check in at the desk, but instead of sitting down in the waiting area, I walk into the intravenous room uninvited and unceremoniously plunk myself down in a large arm-chair. The nurses come up to me very annoyed at me for barging in, but before they can say anything I say, I just got out of the hospital yesterday, I'm so tired I can't even sit up, yes, I was here for over six weeks, I just had a transplant, and I feel so terrible. And then I burst into tears. The head nurse scans the floor, says we have a bed over here in the corner, would you like to lie down? Yes, please.

I slip off my shoes, flop down on the bed, turn my face to the wall, and cry some more. Maybe I left too soon. I'm very discouraged that I have run out of steam so fast on this, my first day out of the hospital. J comes over and sits on the edge of the bed, gives me a lopsided encouraging smile. I think my disintegration has scared him. I'll be okay, J, I just have to rest, why don't you see if you can find a *New York Times* for me outside in the machines?

We read the paper together, then the nurse comes over with the intravenous hookup. Dr. Anderson says your platelets are borderline, and he wants to give you a platelet transfusion, so we'll hook up the IV and give you some normal saline while we wait for the platelets to be ready.

Sounds good to me, maybe part of my problem is dehydration, not getting enough fluids in.

Ken comes by while I'm getting the platelet transfusion. He is all smiles and encouragement, as usual. Yes, he does think I should go ahead and get the second Hickman catheter pulled this afternoon as scheduled. No, I don't have to come back to the hospital again untill Tuesday, I can stay in the apartment, go for walks, and rest.

I go back to the apartment and rest for a couple of hours until it's time to leave for my second outing of the day. Again a short taxi ride, and a longer walk than I can comfortably manage to get to Chip Moore's office. There is an old-fashioned hard wooden bench outside in the main corridor; that is the waiting room. The elderly lady who is waiting there is very nice, and she readily makes room for me so I can lie down on the bench, saying she just got out of the hospital a couple of weeks ago herself and remembers how tired she was.

While Chip Moore removes the second Hickman catheter, again local anesthetic, pulling and tugging, he comments that he never used to take these lines out, five or six years ago. Oh, really, why not? He grimaces slightly, says, They didn't get better. He goes on, The use of these monoclonal antibodies is probably the single greatest clinical application of basic science that I've seen in my lifetime. It works, it makes sense intellectually, and the proof to me is that I'm taking these lines out of people now, and they're recovering fully. Yeah, it is really neat, isn't it? I feel cheered up by Chip's observation, particularly in view of my discouragment this morning. It's good to hear that people do recover, maybe I will too. Of course I will.

Soon after J and I get back to the apartment, Jim arrives with a big smile and a reassuring hug. The problem in New York has been nearly solved, and I am very relieved. He and J trudge off soon to the supermarket for supplies beyond the availabilities of the small market downstairs.

We're here to stay for a while, and we need stuff, I guess, but it's too hard for me to think about, and I am glad that Jim is here to cope.

When Jim returns, I give him the sheets of paper listing all kinds of precautions and dangers to avoid, signs and symptoms of disease I must not ignore. Felice, the transplant nurse, has given all of this to me and included a cute little cartoon from a Swedish advertisement for condoms on the page that details my increased risk for type II herpes and their recommendation that transplant patients use condoms, even monogamous couples. We laugh, they can't be serious!

No raw fish, that includes oysters, for a year. Wash vegetables, salad greens, peel fruit. Stay away from crowds for a while, like a month or two. Avoid restaurants; little lure there, the last thing I can imagine right now is sitting around getting exhausted, waiting for food I don't want and can't taste.

I must report any fever or rash immediately, it's likely to be shingles, old chicken pox revived in the form of herpes zoster, and requires immediate hospitalization for intravenous acyclovir, the medicine I already received for three weeks to decrease the risk of my getting any kind of herpes during the post-transplant time. Shingles could become life-threatening as disseminated chicken pox, especially lethal when it infects the brain of an immune-compromised patient. Still not past the hurdles.

On a more mundane note, I have to throw away all my makeup and buy new stuff (old makeup harbors bacteria). What a waste of good Clinique. I decide to buy new stuff, but not to throw away the old stuff. Maybe I'll do that next Tuesday, when we make another trip to the hospital for blood tests, to see if I need anymore transfusions. Right now I could care less about makeup.

On Thursday morning Jim urges me to get dressed to go out, Come on, let's take a little walk, while the weather's still nice. I put on the same clothes, and my running shoes, and Jim takes my arm. Stop looking at your feet! I know, it's silly, but it doesn't feel right to look ahead, I might trip and fall. I can tell I'm walking like a little old lady, but I can't seem to help it.

We go to the small stream across the street that divides Brookline from Boston. Ducks are swimming there in the turgid water and scuttle to our side when they spy us, hoping we brought something for them. Next time, let's feed the ducks. We sit for a few minutes in the sun on a bench. I think I've had enough, I say. Maybe next time we'll go to the next bench, just a little farther.

In the ensuing days, Jim looks after me assiduously, preparing small meals, dragging me outside once, often twice a day for progressively longer walks. I'm mean and nasty, complain constantly about the unrelenting nausea, with occasional crescendoes of vomiting. This is hardly better than the hospital. I don't understand why I'm still so sick, and I feel very sorry for myself. I want to go back to New York, but I realize that short of a *Star Trek* transporter, there's no way I could make the trip yet. I'm stuck here till I'm strong enough to travel, even if I didn't have to stick around in case I need more platelet or red cell transfusions next week.

Jim sits in the apartment with me, reads and handles problems at the office with long telephone calls. I feel bad that he's enmeshed here as my keeper, and I know I'm no fun to be around, in my black mood of self-pity.

On Sunday we have a very adventuresome trip to the duck stream. As we enter the area, the peace and tranquility is shattered by loud rock music from a ghetto blaster. The noise is so loud that I am tempted to complain to the owner of the box, but the angry look on his face silences me immediately. Jim and I exchange annoyed glances, and I look over at the jerk with the radio again and see the gun. Jim, he's got a gun! Sure enough, the guy is loading a gun. We escape behind the stone wall by the train stop, then we hear shots. Jim hops up on the wall and peers over. He's shooting at the ducks, poor defenseless fat little ducks, almost tame and used to being fed bread crumbs by passersby.

We report the incident to the doorman, who immediately calls in to the police. I feel shaken by the realization of external danger. I have been living with an internal threat for so long that I have forgotten about other calamities, people running amok, car wrecks, plane crashes.

On Tuesday Jim takes me to see Ken in the clinic. My blood tests are fine, white count up to 3000, 40 percent polys, which means 1200, way above the safe level. Too many of those little babies to name now, I think. No need for more transfusions of platelets or red blood cells. If you stay stable all week you should be able to return to New York this weekend, Ken offers. He is very pleased with my progress. I am not. If I'm doing so well, why do I feel so terrible? I feel nauseated all the time, I'm still throwing up, I can hardly walk any distance at all, and I'm very depressed. Ken counters, You maintained your weight this week, that's good. He and Jim agree that I'm being impatient, that it will just take time to feel better, that I should try to get out more, it will come, truly. My gloom is pervasive, unassuaged by their cheerful determination.

On the way home I stop in the drugstore to replace my makeup supplies. Maybe I'll feel better if I get back into the little bit of makeup I used to use. We call this "the lipstick sign": when we come into a patient's room and the lipstick is on, it's a sign that the patient is ready to return to the real world, ready to give up the sick role.

My mother calls to say she is in bed with a bad cold and better not come up as planned for a while. Of course, please don't come up, you sound terrible and probably feel awful too. She'll come later in the week, has to in fact, because she has accumulated a mass of belongings in the apartment that we are about to vacate. It would be nice if she could take some of my stuff back to Litchfield herself, then we'll have less stuff to drag back on the plane ourselves on Saturday when, maybe, we can leave for home.

Friday's visit with Ken at the clinic shows a further increase in my white count, stable hematocrit and platelet count, no weight loss. Ken is very pleased, says I'm ready to go home. Although you were in the hospital much longer than we anticipated, your overall time up here in Boston is about what we figured it would be, so you've really done very well. He beams. I don't think you're going to need any more transfusions at all. You should go see Anne Moore on Monday or Tuesday, I'll call her today and let her know what's happening. Oh, she knows, I say, I've been talking to her every week or so.

When do I have to come back up here? We'd like to get a marrow three months after the transplant, so that would be mid-May sometime. Okay. I cringe at the thought of another bone marrow, but I'm very curious about what it will show. No plasma cells, I hope. When can I go back to work? I ask this almost academically, it's obvious it won't be soon. Let's see how you do, maybe six or eight weeks.

On Saturday we take the late morning shuttle, carrying only a couple of duffel bags. My mother's car has been packed with the rest of the junk I took to the hospital and never used. Mother had argued that we should rent a car and drive down instead of flying. No, I say, that's a four-hour drive, that's much too long for me, if we take the shuttle it's two hours, door to door.

The flight turns rough as we approach LaGuardia. The captain announces we have to circle a bit, there's a severe storm below. The plane bucks wildly, there is silence aboard, passengers stop reading and grip the seat handles. I think this can't be happening, we can't crash now, just when I've gotten this far, we have to find out if the treatment worked. After a half hour of buffeting, the captain announces we have been rerouted to Washington, D.C., to wait out the storm. I hope we won't have to wait long, I feel very tired already.

After a brief while on the ground in Washington we are asked to get off the plane, we will be loaded on the next shuttle to New York, whenever that is. There is a large, confused crowd of stranded travelers already waiting for the next shuttle. It will be at least an hour, we are told. Jim and I get some lunch and return to the waiting area. After another hour, I am feeling totally exhausted, and I go to the check-in counter and explain that I'm just out of the hospital, don't feel well at all, and need a place to lie down. The woman is apologetic, their usual place is being renovated, the only place I could go is the staff smoking lounge, which has chairs like these but no couch to lie down on. No thanks. I return to my seat, lean on Jim's shoulder.

A little later, the service representative approaches me. I know you are not feeling well, she says. I look at her blankly, Yes, that's true. Come with me, there's a place around the corner here that's more quiet, with some open floor space, and I can get you some pillows and blankets and you can lie down and rest. It'll be a couple of hours, we think, before LaGuardia will be open. You are very kind, I say, I'd appreciate that very much. I follow on shaky legs and bed down on the floor with my winter coat and several pillows and blankets.

I lie on the floor and think about how I look to others, huddled on the floor under my coat and blankets, suddenly a homeless person. I feel disconnected and remote and wonder if that's how the people who sleep in subways or out on the street near heating exhausts feel as they regard the people out there, coming and going, engaging in real life. Jim sits near me, and I am comforted by his presence. What about the people who have no one to care for them and are as vulnerable as I?

My rescuer returns to say they will preboard us now, and I follow her, threading my way through a large crowd lined up in anticipation of the call to board. I am grateful that I don't have to stand in line, I know I couldn't do it. The second flight is smooth, and we land in a glorious sunset at LaGuardia. New York has been scrubbed clean by this spring squall, the air is fresh with the promise of spring, the light golden yellow. I'm home.

When we arrive at the apartment, I check my watch. Eight hours, door to door. I laugh at the irony; I guess Mother was right, I should have gone by car. Actually, I should have listened to the weather report, but we were so intent on getting me home at last that I'm not sure we would have postponed the trip by a day if we had known there would be severe wind and rain in New York.

Being home feels so natural, I walk around the apartment despite my fatigue, cloaking myself in familiar surroundings. It's been two months, but all is the same, including the messy desk and bureau, piles of catalogues and magazines in the bedroom, surely they are out of date enough to throw out unread by now. Well, maybe I'll get around to it next week.

APRIL 1987

Unstructured time, time to do all those things I have no time for when I'm working: go to museums, have tea with a friend, walk in the park, read the paper cover to cover, do some professional reading, finish the needlepoint pillows I started in the hospital. The possibilities seem endless as I sit in the empty apartment after Jim has left for the day at seven. My first priority is to get my strength back, so I climb into my sweats and running shoes and walk. For now I'll go around the block, later I'll try to get to Central Park. I walk slowly, and reward myself on my return by buying the paper. I could get it delivered, but I suspect if I did that I might not be motivated to get outside at all.

By the time I return to the apartment I am exhausted. I go back to bed to doze for a while, I'm too tired to sit up. I realize now that unstructured time is of little use when there is no energy with which to use it. I have to ration my events and outings like a miser, no more than one a day.

After a couple of days at home, I mobilize myself for a trip to the office, my work of the day. I get the car out, dusty and unused for two months, and drive myself along the familiar route to the office, get a parking spot only a half block away, luckily. Wouldn't want to exhaust myself just getting there. When I arrive, I meet Drew in the outer hallway, and he gives me a big, uncharacteristic bear hug. It's been so long, he says. Yeah, but I made it. I never doubted you would, he says, but the tears in his eyes belie his words. Before I can get my coat off, he drags me in to see the new office space we just bought to expand into, apologizing for the lack of electricity and consequent darkness. Fiske finds us in the dark there, more hugs and welcome. I beg off on the tour, say I have to sit down and we retreat to my office in the back and chat for a while. Bill finds us there, gives me a crushing hug, comments, You're nothing but bones. That's okay, I laugh, one of the few good things about this is the weight loss. In a while I go to the main office and greet all the secretaries, find George and Charlie seeing patients in back. Everyone's delight and relief at seeing me is apparent and heartwarming. No amount of time on the telephone could equal the in-the-flesh demonstration that I survived, and look well. You look great is the common refrain. I look better than I feel, and soon after lunch and going over some of my mail, I drive home and crawl into bed to rest.

That was a major outing. It is also a little test for myself of how soon I might think about going back to work. I concede to myself that I'm a long way away from actually seeing patients, which involves a fair amount of standing and walking around the office.

Friends come to see me, readily accommodate my inability to travel far without exhaustion and my reluctance to venture out to a public restaurant, even if it's nearby. A visit or lunch is tiring, and I schedule these events sparingly.

A trip to Anne's office is an ordeal, and I soon negotiate the shorter trip to a nearby medical lab for the frequent blood counts, the results of which are discouraging to me, but pleasing to my doctors. My white count is steadily rising, but my hematocrit is worse, dropping a point or two a week. Ken explains this is normal, the old red cells are dying, and they're not being replaced as fast because the regenerating cells are so young. No need to transfuse me now, it's okay if I drift down to 27, could go a lot lower without concern at this point. The platelets are holding with no need for a transfusion, another good sign of a normal regenerating post-transplant marrow. I am right on schedule. Then why am I still so tired? Don't worry, it will come, it will come. You'll see.

I spend time at home on the telephone, organizing the surprise birthday celebration for J's godfather that Jim and I are giving with four other couples, the party we all planned way back in January. I am convinced that by mid-May I should have the energy to go to the party, and the others involved are very interested and cooperative. We divide the tasks: so-and-so will do the flowers, I've reserved the band and arranged the barn on my family's property, another woman and I work out the caterer and the menu with liberal assistance from one of the men, who will get the wine too. We all work on the guest list of fifty people. Someone else does the invitations and I address them, and two couples work out the bar. I do the seating after lengthy consultations with the others. The one who did the invitations will also do the place cards, her penmanship is like calligraphy. I'll go up to Litchfield a day or two before to oversee things with the woman who's doing the flowers. Working on this project is fun, and a welcome focus of my intermittent energy, and not really very much work for me. I am a good delegater, and the others are very cognizant of my infirmity and eager to volunteer. I suspect I am taking unfair advantage of them.

Day by day I increase the length of my morning walk, and by late April I enjoy the flowering trees along the reservoir in Central Park, the crisp wind scattering the petals along the muddy path like confetti. I walk to the lab for my blood tests now, and one day, having rested for twenty minutes waiting to be tested in the lab, I extend my walk through the park at 72nd Street and walk all the way to the office. I am elated by this sign of improvement and set a date for my return to limited office hours: May 18, the Monday after the surprise birthday party. I'll see patients for two to three hours, three or four days a week. I'd much rather spend my energy on seeing patients than going to museums or shopping. I want to get back to my real life.

Abruptly, I feel lousy while I sit waiting for my blood tests on April 29. A queasy malaise overcomes me, and instead of walking home, I grab a taxi, go home and lie down. The ensuing days offer no improvement. Indeed, I find my stamina is decreasing, and depression overwhelms me. I am worse, instead of getting better I'm getting worse. I begin to think I was premature in thinking I could get back to work by mid-May. Relax, you're pushing yourself too hard, just take it easy, it will come. Easy for others to say.

Although I have the disquieting conviction that something is wrong, my malaise is so nonspecific I can't ascribe it to anything more serious than an absurd, dispirited sulk. I'm being a bad sport again. I should be feeling grateful that my marrow has come back so well, that I am ostensibly cured, although it will be some months before the tests can show what I believe is true. Instead I ruminate on my ruined health, wallow in self-pity, and question the wisdom of my decision to go for this cure. Out of the hospital for over a month now, and I'm feeling worse. Could I have gotten AIDS?

By the second weekend in May, driving to Litchfield is so tiring that I have to lie down in the back seat. We have to go, J has the lead in a musical at school and would be crushed if we didn't see his performance. Jim's sister Betsy has driven down from Boston to see the play also and is staying with us for the weekend. I am too bushed to talk to her and retreat to the living room sofa to rest before we go to the performance. Very rude on my part, I know, but I just want to be left alone, conversation is too hard to manage.

The musical comedy is amusing, and J plays his role very well indeed, but I am only too anxious to get away, home and to bed. The next day we leave for New York early, and I watch the baseball game from bed. Suddenly I am shivering with cold. No, Jim says, it's not cold in here, just the opposite, in fact. I find the thermometer, I've got a fever of close to 101. So that's it! I've been sick, not indulging in sulks. The malaise of the last two weeks has some basis in reality. I'm almost relieved.

I catch Anne at home at her country place. We go over my symptoms, nothing but dense fatigue, general malaise, and escalating depression, and now fever, with some joint aches and this shaking chill. No, no headache, gastroenteritis, urinary tract symptoms, sore throat, nothing at all. Let's keep an eye on it, I better see you tomorrow, Anne says. Take some Tylenol. Okay.

Snuggled under my blankets, I note a sharp, sticking pain in my upper left abdomen, under the ribs. Uh-oh, my spleen, something's wrong with my spleen. I reach under my shirt, exhale and relax my stomach to see if I can feel it; if I can, then it's enlarged, maybe I have mono. It's tender, but on the surface, and I think I feel something rough on the skin. Strange. I get up, remove my shirt, go into the bathroom to look in the mirror. Small pink patches about one half inch in diameter. Hey, Jim, lookit this. He agrees, it's faint, but there's something there. I twist around to look at my back, yes, more of them, slanting upward to end at my spine, level with my shoulder blade.

Shingles! I know it instantly and spend the next ten minutes trying to argue myself out of the diagnosis, unsuccessfully. Shingles to lay people, herpes zoster in medical lingo, is a recrudescence of chicken pox, a virus that never leaves the body after that initial childhood infection but lies dormant in the nerve tissue along the spine, the dorsal root ganglia, and can flare up when the immune system is stressed or incompetent. I'm certainly a set-up for that, and indeed I have been warned to be on the lookout for it. But fever and chills and malaise, that's not what I've seen when I've diagnosed zoster in my patients. Usually it starts as nerve-root pain, with the skin lesions appearing a few days later.

I know I have to be hospitalized, and soon. The literature I got when I left Dana-Farber made it very clear that intravenous acyclovir should be started right away to prevent a dangerous dissemination of the virus, which could infect the brain, cause a fatal encephalitis. Shingles is not a dangerous illness for people with intact immune systems, but bone marrow transplant patients are severely compromised for many months following the transplant, until all the young cells have matured into normal function. I have not come this far to take any chances now.

I call Anne again, no answer; on her way to town, no doubt. I call Ken, and he agrees with my diagnosis. Should I come up to Boston, or can I be treated in New York? It's up to you. I think about the trip to Boston. I feel too lousy to travel if I don't have to, I'd rather stay in New York.

When I reach her, Anne tells me to meet her in the emergency room tonight. I pack a bag and carry my pillows—I know better than to expect any decent pillows in the hospital—check in at the ER at my old hospital, familiar after working there for thousands of hours on various rotations. The staff is all changed, no one I remember at all. I know the staff takes a dim view of "the suitcase sign," the patient who arrives with a packed bag, anticipating an admission to the hospital. The ER staff see themselves as handling real emergencies, not patients who should be admitted through the admitting office in regular hours. People like me make unnecessary work for them, and here I am with my suitcase, and pillows too. What a pain! On top of that, I give the nurse my diagnosis as the chief complaint—herpes zoster affecting the left thoracic 8 and 9 dermatomes—and she has trouble with the spelling. She retaliates, however, by giving me an egg-size bruise when she draws my bloods.

Anne agrees with the diagnosis, although she admits she's never seen the skin lesions so early, faint and pale pink blotches. We consult with Ken by phone, make sure of the dosage of acyclovir they give post-transplant patients, somewhat more than is usual. Ken volunteers that twenty percent of the autologous bone marrow transplant patients develop shingles in the first year after the transplant, but I'm a little ahead of schedule, no one has come down with it at three months. I wonder if that's a good sign or not.

Back in a small hospital room again. Not only that, I'm on isolation, too. I'm bummed, to say the least. The fever and chills last another two days, and the skin lesions advance to the blistered stage. I lobby for release from the hospital in time for the party we're giving for our friend on Saturday. It may be possible, if the fever goes away and the skin lesions dry up; after five days of intravenous treatment I could switch to oral acyclovir.

From my hospital room, I delegate the last-minute party details I was going to do myself. My mother takes on overseeing the final preparation of the barn, one woman comes to the hospital to pick up the seating plan, and another covers the rest of the bases. All is set, whether I can make it or not.

The food in the hospital is inedible, except for breakfast. Anne helps me solve that problem by ordering a deli sandwich for me, which is delivered to her third-floor office in the hospital, just down the corridor and around the corner from my room. She brings it over and we have lunch together daily, talk about the commencement address she will be giving to the eighth-grade class of the school our sons attended. I save half my pastrami sandwich for dinner. Given my lack of appetite, it's plenty of food for me.

By Thursday I feel well for the first time since late April. No more fever, but a strong case of cabin fever. I agitate more strongly than ever for a Saturday morning escape from the hospital and enlist the support of the infectious disease specialist Anne has called in consultation. The skin lesions are drying up, and the situation looks good for switching over to oral treatment.

Jim picks me up at the hospital on Saturday, having packed what I need for the weekend, and we drive directly to Litchfield. It's a lovely May day, perfect for the party. Mother has done a wonderful job on the barn, everything is all set. All I have to do is rest.

The secret has been well kept. I had called our friend a couple of weeks ago to tell him dinner would be black tie, as a special celebration of my recovery, with two other couples. When he arrives at our house for dinner, Jim and I tell him of the surprise, and we drive down the road to the barn. He is truly dumbfounded as he walks into the barn to be greeted by his family and close friends, nearly fifty altogether. The party is a tremendous success, the caterer does a fabulous job, music, flowers, food, and wine are all splendid. My energy level is high, and I stay till the party is over, nearly midnight, even dance a little.

I take the acyclovir pills on schedule, but by Sunday night, when I have another shaking chill and the fever is back, I realize I'm having a relapse. No, not again. Maybe I'll be better tomorrow. Not much, the fever is down, but I have new skin lesions surrounding the old crusted ones. Anne is away, so I put a call in to the infectious disease specialist. No response. I call Ken, he agrees I'm having a relapse and need the intravenous treatment again, probably for another week. Does it have to be in the hospital, can I stay home if I can get IV treatment at home? That would be okay, I think.

I sit and stew for a while. I can't face the prospect of another week in isolation in the hospital, I've been hospitalized for over two months this year already. I call the office of a friend who does infectious disease at Roosevelt Hospital and find out which outfit they like the best for home intravenous care. It has suddenly occurred to me that it is not for nothing that I have a medical license: I can order my own intravenous treatment.

I call the home IV people, and they take the order and, more important, my insurance information and say they will call me back. Yes, the wallet biopsy. They call back soon, You have excellent coverage, when would you like to start? As soon as possible. Well, we have to order your supplies from the pharmacy, how about tomorrow morning? Fine. Later in the evening, the infectious disease guy calls me back, and I tell him I've arranged for home IV treatment. Good. You probably ought to stay on it for another full week to be on the safe side this time, we really don't know a whole lot about zoster in your situation, usually the oral treatment is all we use.

A cheerful nurse arrives first thing in the morning and starts the heparin lock, an intravenous line that is "locked" with heparin to keep it from clotting off when fluid is not running through. With a heparin lock, I'll be free of the IV pole except when the dose is running in, three times a day. While she is there, the supplies are delivered, and she shows me how to mix and label the doses day by day, how to flush the line with heparin solution to keep it open.

What an improvement over being in the hospital! I still feel lousy, still have a fever, but being at home is infinitely better. I can even go outside to get the paper. Why didn't I think of this last week? In three days the fever is gone, and I feel well again. I complete the week of intravenous acyclovir anyway. I call my secretary and tell her I'll start seeing patients June 1.

On May 28 I fly to Boston for a bone marrow, the three-month checkup we had to postpone when I was in the hospital with shingles. It's great to see Ken again, and I am welcomed warmly by the nurses in the clinic who remember me from last winter. After the marrow, before leaving, I go upstairs to my old floor and find a few of the nurses who cared for me. They are delighted to see me looking well, say it boosts their morale to see that their patients do recover.

JUNE AND JULY 1987

Office hours on Monday. After four months of being unable to work, it's wonderful to see patients again, so natural that I feel almost as if I had never been away. Some of my old patients inquire politely about my sabbatical, did I learn a lot? Yes, it was—interesting, I allow. I limit myself to just a few hours a day for the first week, stop my walks, reserve my energy for work. My highest priority is to get back to a full schedule, and to start operating again.

Ken calls with good news about the bone marrow. A totally normal regenerating marrow, no evidence of abnormal plasma cells at all. I think I'm cured, I tell him. Yes, it looks very good. What about the protein electrophoresis, what does that show? Well, ours isn't back yet, but I just got a copy from Anne of the one they did when you were in the hospital three weeks ago. And? The quantities are normal, the curve is normal, but there is still a notation that an abnormal protein is present, just as it was in March when you left the hospital.

We discuss this some more, consider the life span of the abnormal protein that I had circulating at the start of my treatment. Given that the half-life of the immunoglobulin molecule is about one month, it is possible that the ones that are abnormal are still circulating from before the treatment, three months before. None of the treatment was directed at the proteins themselves, only at the cells that produced them. No need, therefore, to be discouraged that the protein electrophoresis is not totally normal yet, it may be too soon.

We hang up, and I think some more about the protein electrophoresis test. Although we talk about an abnormal protein, we know the protein itself is not abnormal, it's the fact that it is present in a larger amount that's notable. The electrophoresis test is a very sensitive marker for an abnormal amount of a molecule of a certain weight, because each globulin has a slightly different structure and molecular weight. The test is done by placing a small amount of the serum protein in an agar gel and running an electric charge through it that draws the molecules through the resistance of the gel, like a magnet pulling iron filings. The molecules hang up in the gel at various points, depending on their molecular weight. If a whole bunch of molecules are the same weight, they all pile up on the same line, instead of being dispersed throughout the gel as a heterogeneous assortment would be. Thus, even when the amount of protein is normal, a signature of an abnormal identical clone of immunoglobulin remains in the gel because too many molecules wind up at the same spot, instead of being evenly distributed throughout the gel.

Ever since protein electrophoresis was discovered, it has been known that some few people produce a monoclonal protein, an M protein, or M spike, in a small amount, and this condition is called benign monoclonal gammopathy, or BMG. With repeat electrophoresis over time, many of these people continue to have an M protein that stays stable, and they remain totally healthy. Some, however, go on to develop myeloma with a large amount of M protein, and bone marrows that reveal too many plasma cells, 15 percent or more, compared to the 2 to 5 percent plasma cells found in normal bone marrow.

It is not really known what distinguishes people who have a benign monoclonal gammopathy from those who will eventually develop myeloma, nor is it known how long a period of time is involved for myeloma to develop in any particular person. In my own case, for instance, there may have been a time when I had no M protein, and that might have been in childhood, or my teens, or early adulthood. At some point, the monoclonal cells producing my M protein blasted off, and I wound up finding myself with advanced myeloma when I first learned I had the disease a year ago. But the hallmark of multiple myeloma is too much of one particular immunoglobulin, and I would rather have no M protein at all.

I know that the original protocol did not list a normal protein electrophoresis as a criterion for cure. A normal marrow and reconstitution of the marrow were the goals set forth. And I remember that Anne had told me that the identical twin transplant done about seven years ago had not eliminated the abnormal protein, although the twin had remained disease free all these years.

But in my own mind, a normal protein electrophoresis is my goal. That would mean that all the cells of the malignant clone are gone—an outward and visible sign of a cure. The six-month checkup will be very key because by then the half-life of the protein I had in January should be exhausted, and if the protein electrophoresis is normal, I'll feel that we have a cure.

Meanwhile, it's back to real life, day-to-day recovery. Although the skin lesions from the shingles have cleared, leaving a broad, three-inch welt of flat, dark scars on my skin from my spine around my ribs to my midline in front, the nerve root, a sensory one, which was infected by the virus, is hypersensitive, and very painful. It is getting worse every day, wakes me at night when I move in my sleep. Shingles is known to be a very painful affliction, and I had been somewhat surprised and relieved that I had no pain all during May when I was systemically sick. Now we're making up for that, I conclude.

I get by on Tylenol, stronger narcotic pain medicine doesn't help, only makes me feel loopy. Charlie Goodwin suggests I consult with a pain management specialist who has helped a number of his patients. I am worried because the pain is getting worse every day, and I know that some people, only a small percent, to be sure, develop very severe and unremitting chronic pain as a sequela of herpes zoster.

I go see the pain specialist. He is a young anesthesiologist who devotes all of his practice to pain management, rather than giving anesthesia to patients undergoing surgery. He suggests that one or two steroid and local anesthetic injections around the affected nerve root may tone down the inflammation causing the symptoms, and he also advises a short course of Elavil, a common antidepressant medicine that has been found to damp down hyperactive peripheral nerves long before any central or emotional effect would be noted. After two injections and a week of Elavil, the pain is gone.

My stamina increases rapidly as the pain diminishes, I increase my office hours, and plan to start operating in July. I send a letter concerning my recovery and return to work to the colleagues who had received my letter announcing my leave of absence, and soon I receive many congratulatory letters and phone calls, and referrals of patients who had been waiting for my return.

More seemingly trivial aspects of normal life emerge, what I used to take for granted, but lost for so long I thought I'd never get them back. My sense of taste gradually comes back four months after the radiation therapy, the culprit that eliminated my taste for most foods. Normal saliva production returns, too, and I can now eat without using milk to wash everything down.

Now that the salivary glands have recovered from the effects of radiation, I should have normal tear fluid levels to allow me to wear contact lenses again. No problem, says the ophthamologist after he measures my tear fluid production on special blotting paper. Go ahead and get new lenses. The old ones don't fit anymore. With my lenses, I begin to look like my old self again.

I still have to wear my wig, though. It's hot and uncomfortable, and I wish I could be done with it, but all I have is about a half inch of what appears to be ash brown hair. Jim asserts the gray is gone. That's too good to be true, it's just too short for us to see it yet, I predict. One Saturday morning I rush out of the apartment building to get the paper in the machine on the corner, and a huge gust of wind blows the wig off my head and sends it rolling along the sidewalk like a tumbleweed. I race after it, grab it, and plunk it back on my head, then look around to see if anyone else is around. No, no one. Whew! I am so rattled by this worst nightmare of wig wearing that I put my coins in the newspaper machine before I notice it's empty. Soon, though, the incident seems more comical than embarrassing, particularly because New York apartment dwellers cloak themselves in protective anonymity, I among them, and if I was seen, it wouldn't be as if anyone knew who I was, I could be any crazy bald woman, you see everything in New York.

AUGUST 1987

I board the shuttle for Boston on August 12, almost a year to the day from my first trip to Dana-Farber, when I was desperate for a cure of my fatal illness. I'm anxious, to say the least, about these tests. What if it didn't work, can I stand to find out that it didn't work after all? My former life has been restored to me, and I feel profoundly grateful. Will I lose it again?

Ken greets me with an affectionate hug, we are old friends now. He is amazed, I can tell, at the transformation of my looks. You never saw my real hair color before, you know, Ken; it was dyed last year, now it's come back the color it was ten years ago, all the gray is gone, and it's got all this curl! I tug at my ringlets with glee. See, this is the real thing. Ken laughs with me in delight. But, I add ruefully, my appetite has really returned and now I'm gaining weight. That's okay, you're entitled.

I fill him in on my activities. I'm back to a regular schedule at work, and I'm operating a couple of days a week. I'm tired at the end of the day, and I haven't started exercising yet, I'm going to wait a while more and see how my energy level is. Very good, Ken says, beaming. Last month we went to Santa Fe for some meeting, and I gave some talks, and Jim's going to take a few days off next month and we'll go to Oakland, where I'm going to give a couple of talks at a teaching course, and while we're out there we'll tour the wine country for a couple of days. Then in November I go to San Diego for a few days to be on the faculty of another course for orthopaedic surgeons, that should be fun because I've never been there before. And in December we're going to go to Vail for a week of skiing and meetings. Whew, Ken says, I don't know where you get all your energy. I've always had a lot of energy, I'm just now getting it back.

You know, I'm still not taking call to the emergency room, is that still the rule? Yeah, I think that would be better, till your immune system has had a chance to mature. Our other patients generally don't reconstitute the subtle parts of their immune response till about a year after the transplant, so it would be better if you avoid having to operate on patients who may have diseases you may not be able to defend against too well right now. Okay, then, I'll wait till the year is up.

How are the troops? Ken asks. How is Jim doing, your chief coach? Oh, Jim is great, things are going very well at work now for him, over the next few months he's going to be finishing up some current project, and then he's going to create a whole new role for himself, coordinating his agency's media department's use of computer systems. He's really excited about it, it's going to be very interesting, and uniquely suited to his talents.

And the kids? How are Heather and J? They're fine, too. Heather went to Europe for a month when she got out of school in May, visited some friends and also traveled around on her own. She found out what I could have told her, that it's more fun being with people you know than traveling around strange places all by yourself. She's been at home with us since June, working at an office job, and seeing what it's like to be a yuppie in the city. It seems to have gotten her motivated to work hard in school, she's quite ambitious.

And J just got back from a group trip to Spain with a bunch of teenagers and a group leader, they spoke only Spanish and lived for a while with a Spanish host family. He's taking advanced-placement Spanish next year and wanted to get fluent. I think he had a good time, he certainly looks great, even taller and thinner and very tanned.

By now it's bone marrow time, ugh. I notice the technician is setting up for two marrows; when Ken comes into the room, I accost him. What's this? I thought we were just doing one side. Well, the protocol actually calls for bilateral iliac crest biopsies. Yes, I remember, but I think it's ridiculous, you'll get all the information you need from one side. Okay, Ken agrees reluctantly, if you really don't want to, we won't. I feel mean-spirited and selfish. This is the last time we're going to do this without general anesthesia. Let's see how the first one goes, then we'll see. Ken puts in the local anesthetic, I can still feel it. Try putting in the rest of the bottle, use the whole thirty cc. Okay. That's better, not so bad. All right, you can do the other side, but use the whole bottle. At last, it's over. Now I can enjoy the rest of the day.

In a few minutes I get large quantities of peripheral blood drawn for the other tests—the routine CBC, blood chemistries, and serum protein electrophoresis require only small tubes, but the complex immunologic analyses require large syringes of blood. These samples will be used to determine the populations of white cells that have reconstituted since the transplant, what proportion of white cells are natural killer cells, helper cells, suppressor cells, all very interesting from the point of view of the protocol. For me, the only important test is the serum protein electrophoresis. If that reverts to normal, then I will know I am cured.

Ken calls me a couple of days later with the results of the bone marrow—totally normal. I am pleased, of course, but I kind of expected it would be. The CBC is about the same as it has been, low normal hematocrit, slightly less than normal platelet count, but plenty of platelets for my needs, and they seem to be regenerating on the same time frame as other transplant patients'. The serum protein electrophoresis isn't back yet, so we hang up, and I'm still on edge and know I will be till I find out.

I call Ken a week later. Didja get the electrophoresis back yet? Yes, just this morning, as a matter of fact, I was going to call you—it's normal. Really? Yes. No notation about an abnormal protein? No, none. Then I'm cured. Yes, it looks that way. I am flooded with relief, then immediately think, of course, how could I have doubted?

To my knowledge, Ken, correct me if I'm wrong, but this has never been done before, has it? Even the identical twin transplant had an abnormal protein, right? Yes. Wow, I'm so happy, so thrilled! Ken says, Well, I don't know who's happier, you or me. I am, I say emphatically.

You know, Cesca, today I was organizing your chart for the reviewer from the National Institutes of Health who's coming next month, and I really looked at the protein electrophoresis we did when you were here at the end of May, and it was normal too. What? Yes, I didn't pay much attention to it because the one from three weeks before was fresh in my mind. So, I conclude, it reverted to normal at the end of May, I was cured all along and didn't know for sure. Yup. Well, it's great news, even if delayed.

I call Jim right away, tell him of my cure. I knew it, he says, I knew you would be cured. I tell Charlie and George and Drew. Drew says, Of course, I never doubted it would work. How can everyone else be so sure? To me, this is the most amazing result in the treatment of multiple myeloma, an incredible conversion of molecular biological theory to clinical outcome. I guess it's so overwhelming to think of the impossibilities overcome, to encompass the miracle created by Ken and his colleagues, that it's easier to shrug and say, Of course, isn't modern technology elegant, of course it worked, it was a good idea, well executed.

I call Anne, of course, too, and she is very pleased. That's good, Cesca, very good. She's saying the natural things, but she has a tone of voice that is somewhat flat, not totally exhilarated, as I am. I wonder why, but say nothing about it. I think oncologists have a different approach to thinking about cures, one that isn't black and white, more hedged, more cautious.

SEPTEMBER 1987

My friend from residency who called me every night when I was in the hospital comes to Litchfield on Labor Day weekend with his wife and their two babies. This is our first weekend visit since my illness, and as usual our talk is incessant. He brings up the subject of my experience with this illness, do I think I've changed at all? I don't know, I don't have much perspective on it yet, certainly I feel much more identified with people who are sick or disabled, having been so sick myself. I don't think I'll push my patients so hard to get going when they're down and out, the way I used to.

For a while I thought about starting a halfway house for AIDS patients up here in that old barn next door, this would be a beautiful place to stay when you're too sick to live on your own but too well to stay in the hospital. Really? Yeah, but I looked into it some more, and it appears that AIDS patients need much more medical coverage than I had thought, and it would cost about five times more than I would have guessed to make the barn habitable for even healthy people. So I've put that bright idea on hold.

But what about the experience itself, going through the transplant? Well, I'm always embarrassed when people say I was brave to do it. The truth is, I wasn't brave at all. It was very much like someone who's on the fifth floor of a burning building: you can stay in and be a crispy critter, or you can jump into the safety net below. The transplant was the safety net.

I think the hardest part of the whole thing for me was being so aware of how far short of my ideal self I was in all that stress. I've been thinking about that lately, and I recall some other stressful times, like when I was coping with two little babies at home, or when I was an intern. I had this idealized notion that I would be a great mother, warm and giving, and I found myself short of sleep, resentful of incessant demands, even yelling at them, and the most upsetting thing was not living up to that fantasy of myself as the great earth mother. Again, when I was an intern, the work load was enormous, sleep was scant, and I found myself shutting off to my patients just so I could get my work done and then being hard on myself for not living up to my ideal of being a caring, compassionate doc. Looking back on it, I can see now that I was perhaps too hard on myself for feeling like a poor sport all the time when I was sick. Yeah, he says, grinning, maybe you're just human like the rest of us. Yeah.

I guess you could say I have a case of survivor debt. You know, when I was getting myself ready for the transplant, I imagined myself getting cured, and that this cure would be the first of what would become routine for myeloma patients within ten years. I feel very strongly that this treatment shouldn't be just for someone like me, in the medical elite, with special connections. This is a method that works, and it could be applied to many people with myeloma—did you know that ten thousand people a year develop myeloma in this country alone?

You and I were trained to think of myeloma as a fatal disease of old people. Well, it's not just old people, it's young people, too. Now there appears to be a treatment that offers something really substantial compared to routine chemo, and I want other people in my situation to hear about it before their disease progresses too much to have a transplant.

So what are you going to do? I'm going to tell my story, write a book. No kidding, what are you going to call it? I'm calling it *Going for the Cure.*

NOVEMBER 1987

Another three-month checkup in Boston. I should, according to the protocol, be getting another bone marrow, but two weeks ago I went to my own lab for an immunoelectrophoresis, and it was normal. I have it in hand, and I'm going to use it with Ken to argue for a postponement of the bone marrow test till a year after the transplant, and just have all those fancy blood tests of my immune system's recovery from the transplant that are part of the protocol also.

I am very persuasive, Ken agrees to just the blood tests, so the checkup doesn't take long. We have an hour or so before dinner—I'm taking Ken and Karen and Cox out to dinner to celebrate—so Ken and I visit the transplant floor, see some of the nurses and visit for a while.

Where is my other bone marrow harvest kept? I ask Ken. You want to see it? It's right upstairs in the labs. He takes me up to one of the research floors, they far outnumber the two patient treatment floors in this research hospital, and shows me a small room with some large refrigerators. Back in the corner is a stainless steel cannister about the size of a beer keg, and it is under a special alarm mechanism, cooled by tanks of liquid nitrogen to an exceedingly low temperature. That's it, huh?

While we're up here, I can show you where we treated your marrow on the day of your first harvest. Oh, I'd love to see that. The room is tiny, really just a black marble countertop against a wall, with cabinets above and below, like a kitchen, and an overhanging see-through hood. You work with your hands under the hood, which prevents you from breathing on your work area, or breathing fumes from it. Really a standard organic chemistry type of work station. I wonder how they kept it sterile, it's right next to the hallway, no special isolation at all.

We pass by an open office, and Ken stops to show me off to Jerry Ritz. I am glad to have a chance to see him again, he was the attending of the month in March when I was having such a hard time, and he was flogging me to get up and get going. I want him to see me recovered, but I also especially want to thank him directly for having invented one of the antibodies that was used to clean up my marrow. I do, and his response is a good approximation of a John Wayne–type aw, shucks, ma'am, it weren't nothin'. Underneath it, though, I think he is pleased. I would hope he is; there are not many scientific researchers who get to see their work translated into real, meaningful clinical results. I feel profoundly grateful for his work.

Do you suppose Lee Nadler is around? I ask Ken as we move down the hall. I'd like to thank him too. He might be, his office is right here. Lee Nadler invented the first of the three antibodies used to clean up my marrow, and he was the one almost a year ago who called me up to tell me I had to have the second consolidation chemotherapy with the high-dose steroids, so we have talked on the phone, but never met.

He is in his office, tidying up to leave for home. He is happy to meet me and says he's been keeping tabs on me through Ken, but it's great to see me looking so well. I thank him for his part in my treatment, and he is pleased, but he continues to gather up his things as we chat. He apologizes for being rushed, explaining that he promised his fifteen-year-old son that he would review his essay on Shakespeare with him tonight, so he has to rush home now and do that before he goes to his moonlighting job in an emergency room. I am incredulous. You moonlight? Yes. I look at Ken, accusingly, and see him nodding his head, almost sadly. You, too? Yes. Lee Nadler leaves, hustling to be a good father and hold down a second job as well.

I feel humbled, even guilty. These guys have saved my life, and many others as well with their scientific research, but at what personal sacrifice? Ken and I continue on to dinner, and I badger him with questions. Yes, they are on a salary here, but it's not much, not enough to cover the high cost of mortgages in the Boston area and saving for children's college and other educational expenses. I am reminded of the witticism I saw on a cocktail napkin: mid-life crisis is when your mortgage and tuition payments equal more than your salary. Ken knew when he chose academic research instead of private practice that his income would be limited; I wonder if he knew back then what it would mean as far as time spent away from his family, working a second part-time job. I wonder if the thrill of having invented an antibody that has saved someone like me, and potentially may help thousands of others, makes up for his sacrifice.

I want to do all I can to help Ken in his work with myeloma patients. I tell him about the book I am writing, that I will send it to any prospective transplant patients when it's done, but meanwhile, I'd be very happy to talk to any patients who want to talk to me, and he can give them both my home and office numbers, they can call me anytime. Actually, Ken has already given my numbers to a couple of patients who have called me and talked to me at length, and I've even met with them. Ken has seemed apologetic about the intrusion, though, so I want to reiterate that I am very happy to do this. Okay, if you're sure you don't mind, it really helps them a lot.

Soon I have a small group of people, my myeloma club, and they are in various stages of treatment to get ready for the transplant themselves. They keep in touch with me to report on how their treatment is going, what side effects they're experiencing, and how they're keeping up with the rest of their lives. And we talk a lot about what the transplant is like, and how I'm faring now.

FEBRUARY 1988

It's Lincoln's Birthday, the anniversary of my transplant, and again I'm on the way up to Boston. I want to have the bone marrow test on the exact anniversary. My immunoelectrophoresis is still normal, so I expect the marrow will be, too, but it has to be done to report the results to the committees that review experimental research.

It's a busy day. In addition to my tests, I meet a guy I've talked to on the phone many times who is going to have the transplant when he gets into remission. We go out for a beer, and I give him a first draft of my book. He is about forty-two, an astrophysicist, engaged to be married in March, and he has known about his disease for about two years. Last year it started to progress. He is very keen on the transplant, impatient to be ready, but it sounds like it will take him several more months, time enough to get married and have a nice honeymoon first.

When I get back to the hospital Ken takes me upstairs to meet the second myeloma transplant patient, who got his treated cells just the day before. He's fifty-three, works as an office manager, and has had myeloma for about three years, and it took a very long time to get him ready for the transplant. He looks pretty good to me, considering what he's been through this week, but I remember that this is the quiet before the storm of side effects from the treatment. His sore throat and fatigue will probably start on Sunday. We chat briefly, but the most morale-boosting aspect of my visit is how I look to him: healthy, active, vigorous, working full tilt again, skiing again, brimming with energy. And I don't have myeloma anymore. This is what he'll remember when things get tough in the next few weeks.

Before I leave Boston, Ken asks me if I would come up to Boston in April to be the speaker at a brunch the blood component laboratory he directs is giving to honor the people who have made many donations of blood and platelets to the patients at Dana-Farber. They like to see the end result, Ken says, and you are our star patient. Of course, it will be a delight, but I think to myself, what am I going to say, except thanks?

MARCH 1988

We spend nearly three weeks in the Italian Alps, at my family's house, my mother and Jim and J and me, Heather can only spend a week before she has to return to school. It is idyllic. Jim and I ski all morning, sometimes part of the afternoon as well. I read, relax, think about how my life has changed, or has it? Certainly the outward aspects are no different from before my illness—my practice is busy, I love my work, Jim and I are happy together, our lives revolve around each other. Heather and J are open and communicative.

Jim is very relaxed, mellow; now that the crisis is over, I can see the difference in him, the tightness of holding himself together for me has dissipated, he has expanded somehow. Funny I didn't notice it last year. Am I different, too? I feel at ease with myself now, not exactly self-satisfied or smug, but I see myself as good enough, as a mother, a wife, a surgeon, a person, good enough just the way I am, as imperfect as it is. I'm not pissed off at myself. Is this the true gift of the transplant? Have I come out of this a different me?

I ride the chair lift and absorb the mountains, ponder what I can say to the blood and platelet donors. It will be Easter then, early spring. I want to tell them about my illness, and my new life. Oh, well, I can work on it when I get home, leave it on the back burner for now.

APRIL 1988

I go up to Boston with my recent blood test results—
all normal—and my speech synopsized on index cards. I
don't want to forget what I intend to say. There is a crowd
of happy people in the large room on the top floor of Dana-
Farber where the brunch is set up. At each place setting is
a sheet of paper listing the donors by name and number of
donations. Wow! When Ken told me they had some big
givers, I had no idea he was talking about a significant
number of people who have given over a hundred times, a
dozen or so over two hundred times, and one individual
who has made over three hundred donations. I start to calculate how many hours of platelet pheresis three hundred
platelet donations represents, six hundred hours, that's
about twenty-five days of being hooked up to a pheresis
machine. Donations can only be made weekly, so this guy's
been doing this weekly for at least six years. That is some
committment. I'm impressed.

At the end of the meal, after some welcoming
speeches, I am introduced to the group. I tell them a brief
story of my illness, my chemotherapy, my concerns about
safe transfusions, and my transplant and subsequent recovery. I conclude, This is a time of year when we celebrate
new life, resurrection, and renewal. Last week was Easter,
today is Orthodox Easter. It seems entirely fitting to me
that we are gathered together here today to celebrate the

gift of resurrection and new life that you offer to us patients all the year round. Thanks to you, I am the first person to be able to say, I had multiple myeloma, but now I am cured. And thanks to you, more patients will follow, and, in a few years, we'll be able to put multiple myeloma in the cure column. Thank you for making miracles possible.

Everyone has tears in their eyes when I finish, including me. I walk over to Ken. I know it was corny, I say, but I wanted them to really get what a great thing it is that they do. No, it was great. I hope he got the message also, the guy who invents antibodies that save lives, the guy who spends every other Saturday at another job to supplement his low salary.

MAY 1988

Spring progresses, and so does my appreciation of my resurrection, my metamorphosis. I am engulfed in happiness. Every day is great. I'm not living for tomorrow, everything is fine in the moment, the present, the now.

I talk to Jim about this change. Remember how I used to be upset about something that I didn't like about my current circumstances, and I'd look forward to the future, just hang on for something, like, when the kids are out of diapers, things will really be great, or, when I finish medical school . . . or, when I pass my boards . . . or whatever. I was always hanging myself up on some as yet unrealized event, and missing the actual experience of the present. You never did that, I tell him, and now I think I've finally learned how not to do it. Jim smiles, squeezes my hand. I'm no longer waiting for some marvelous thing to happen, it's okay just the way it is right now.

This is going to sound very strange, honey, but sometimes I think maybe this illness is the best thing that ever happened to me. A sharp look. No, I guess really I'd rather not have gone through it, but as mid-life crises go, this was a major one, just like what the family always says about Daddy, he never does things by halves, *il faut toujours qu'il exagère*, in many ways I'm the same way. I still don't know if there is a God, but if there is, he must have thought, Now first, I have to get her attention. Yes, it really got my attention, and I'll never be the same again. A very strange kind of gift.

JUNE 1988

I call in to the lab for my every-other-month lab results. The quantities of the immune globulins are normal, but there is a notation on the immunoelectrophoresis that there is an abnormal protein on the smear. What does this mean? More tests, bone marrows in Boston, special staining. The regular bone marrow is normal, twenty-four of the twenty-five specially stained slides are normal, but on one corner of one slide, a few cells are found that stain all the same way, suggestive of a clone of cells making the same stuff, perhaps the protein that showed up on the electrophoresis.

What does this mean? We don't know, this is totally virgin territory, Ken says. Would you still call it a cure? Look, you don't have myeloma now, you'd have to have a big spike of M protein and at least 15 percent plasma cells in your marrow to make a diagnosis of myeloma. But? But we have to watch it, follow the immunoelectrophoresis, see what happens. So I have a great remission? You have a spectacular remission. No one has had the bulk of disease you had, ninety-five percent of your marrow was tumor when you were first diagnosed, and you've had no treatment for sixteen months now and all you have is a notation of an abnormal M protein in your IgG immunoelectrophoresis, but your marrow is normal, and the other two immune globulins, the IgA and IgM, are normal too. For all we know, it could stay like that for years, until we both grow old and die. But if it doesn't? And if it doesn't, then there's a lot we can do, if you ever get something that needs treatment, but there sure is nothing there to treat now.

I get it. Cure is declared when I grow old and die of something unrelated. I'm still going for the cure.

The author's royalties are being donated to Cure Myeloma Fund, Inc., a New York State tax-exempt not-for-profit corporation.

Contributions are welcome and may be sent to Suite 11, 345 W. 58 St., New York, NY, 10019. Please make checks payable directly to the corporation.